# Sleep well, Live better

## The role of sleep in health and well-being

Julio Rodriguez

## Introduction...........8
### Importance of sleep for physical, mental and emotional health........... 8
- physical benefits of sleep...........8
- Impact of sleep on mental health........... 10
- Influence of sleep on emotional abilities........... 12

### Statistics on sleep problems in today's society.......14
- Prevalence of sleep disorders...........15
- Consequences of sleep deprivation...........18
- Lifestyle and socioeconomic factors related to sleep........... 20

### Purpose of Book: To provide information and strategies to help people sleep better...........23
- Importance of sleep education...........23

## Fundamentals of Sleep........... 28
### The science behind sleep: the circadian cycle, sleep stages and their characteristics........... 28
- the circadian cycle........... 28
- sleep stages...........30
- Functions and benefits of sleep........... 32

### Optimal sleep duration for different age groups......35
- Sleep recommendations by age group........... 35
- Importance of individuality........... 38

### Impact of inadequate sleep on health and well-being. 40
- Consequences of sleep deprivation...........40
- Relationship between sleep and mental health 42
- Importance of quality sleep for overall well-being. 45

**Identifying Sleep Disorders..................... 50**
   Main sleep disorders: insomnia, sleep apnea, narcolepsy, restless legs syndrome, among others 50
      Insomnia................................................................ 50
      Sleep apnea..........................................................53
      narcolepsy.............................................................55
      Restless legs syndrome (RLS)........................ 58
   When to seek specialist medical help....................61
      Recognizing the need for professional assistance.......................................................61
      Health professionals specializing in sleep disorders........................................................... 64
      Available treatments and therapies.................67

**Hygiene do Sono........................................................ 72**
   Establishing a healthy sleep routine: regular schedules, suitable environment, relaxing rituals... 73
      regular hours.......................................................73
      suitable environment.........................................76
      relaxing rituals....................................................78
   The impact of diet and exercise on sleep quality....81
      Food for healthy sleep....................................... 81
      Physical exercise and sleep..............................84
   Managing stress and anxiety before bed................87
      Stress management strategies........................ 87
      Dealing with Nocturnal Anxiety........................ 90

**Improving the Sleep Environment......................... 96**
   Creating an environment conducive to sleep: mattress, pillows, temperature, light and noise.......96
      Choosing the right mattress..............................96

Selecting the Perfect Pillows............................99
Regulating the room temperature.................. 102
Dealing with light and noise........................... 105
The importance of darkness and tips for blocking out excessive light..................................................... 107
The role of darkness in sleep regulation......... 107
Strategies to block out excessive light............ 109
The role of technology in sleep quality: electronic devices, blue light and strategies to minimize its negative impact................................................... 111
Understanding the influence of technology on sleep.................................................................. 111
Strategies to minimize the negative impact of technology on sleep........................................... 114

**Relaxation and Meditation Techniques...................119**
Relaxation practices to prepare the body and mind for sleep............................................................... 119
Hot shower........................................................ 119
Massage............................................................ 120
Stretching and Gentle Yoga.............................. 122
Meditation and mindfulness as tools to reduce anxiety and promote peaceful sleep..................... 125
guided meditation.............................................125
mindfulness practice......................................... 127
Breathing exercises and other techniques to calm the mind before bed............................................. 130
Deep breath...................................................... 130
progressive muscle relaxation......................... 132
guided views.................................................... 135

**Supplements and Natural Remedies...................... 141**

4

Natural alternatives to aid sleep, such as calming teas and essential oils........................................... 141
    calming teas.................................................... 141
    Essential oils.................................................... 144
Dietary supplements that can promote healthy sleep. 147
    Melatonin........................................................ 147
    tryptophan and magnesium........................... 150
Considerations about the use of sleeping pills and their possible consequences............................... 153
    sleeping pills................................................... 154
    Possible consequences of using sleeping pills:.... 156

**Strategies for Different Stages of Life................... 162**
Tips for sleeping well during childhood, adolescence, adulthood and old age......................................... 162
    Infancy............................................................ 162
    Adolescence................................................... 164
    adult life..........................................................166
    Third Age....................................................... 168
Sleep during pregnancy and the necessary care for mothers-to-be........................................................ 170
    Sleep care during pregnancy...........................170
    Preparation for sleep after childbirth............... 172

**Managing Jet Lag and Irregular Timings................178**
Tips for minimizing the effects of jet lag after travel.... 178
    Entendendo o jet lag........................................ 178
    Preparation before the trip............................. 180
    During flight....................................................183

upon arrival..................................................184
Strategies for people who work shifts or have irregular sleep schedules........................................187
   Understanding the challenges of irregular hours.. 187
   Managing irregular hours...............................191
   Health care.....................................................193
How to adjust the internal clock and maintain consistency even under challenging circumstances... 196
   Adjusting the internal clock........................... 196
   Additional Strategies..................................... 199

**I am and Saude Mental..............................................206**
The link between sleep and mental health: How sleep deprivation can affect mood, anxiety and depression........................................................... 206
   Importance of sleep for mental health.............206
   Impact of sleep deprivation on mental health. 208
   cycle of mutual influence................................211
Strategies to improve sleep in cases of mental disorders........................................................... 214
   Identifying and treating comorbid sleep disorders 214
   Adapted sleep hygiene practices....................217
   Cognitive behavioral therapy for insomnia (CBT-I)............................................................. 219
Complementary therapies to promote mental health through sleep....................................................222
   Sono therapy and complementary therapies:. 222

**The Role of the Dream...........................................229**

The importance of dreams for health and emotional processing.......................................................... 229
    understanding dreams.................................. 229
    emotional processing..................................... 231
    adaptive dream function................................ 234
Dream interpretation: psychological and cultural approaches........................................................... 237
    psychological approaches............................. 237
    cultural influence............................................ 240
Techniques for remembering and recording dreams meaningfully........................................................ 242
    Improving dream recall................................... 242
    Exploring and interpreting dreams................. 244
    Incorporating dreams into the personal journey.... 247

**Conclusion............................................................ 253**

# Introduction

*Importance of sleep for physical, mental and emotional health*

A good night's sleep is essential for overall health and well-being. In this section, we will explore the importance of sleep in different aspects of life.

## physical benefits of sleep

Sleep plays a key role in promoting physical health. During sleep, the body goes through a process of restoration and regeneration, allowing the recovery of damaged tissues and cell repair. This process is essential for maintaining health and for the proper functioning of various body systems.

One of the most important physical benefits of sleep is strengthening the immune system. During sleep, the body produces and releases cytokines, proteins responsible for the immune response, which play a crucial role in defending the body against infections and diseases. Sleep deprivation can compromise the effectiveness of the immune system, making the body more susceptible to infections and illnesses.

Furthermore, adequate sleep is directly related to improved cardiovascular function. During sleep, blood pressure decreases, allowing the heart to rest and reducing the workload on the cardiovascular system. Lack of sleep can lead to increased blood pressure and the development of cardiovascular conditions such as hypertension, heart disease and stroke.

Sleep also plays an important role in regulating weight and metabolism. Sleep deprivation can affect the hormones involved in appetite control, leading to imbalances that increase hunger and cravings for high-calorie, unhealthy foods. Furthermore, lack of sleep can affect the regulation of blood glucose levels and insulin sensitivity, increasing the risk of developing type 2 diabetes and obesity.

In short, adequate sleep offers significant physical benefits, including restoring and regenerating the body, strengthening the immune system, improving cardiovascular function, and regulating weight and metabolism. It is essential to prioritize healthy sleep as part of a balanced lifestyle to promote health and physical well-being.

## Impact of sleep on mental health

Sleep plays a crucial role in mental health and emotional well-being. Good quality sleep is directly related to a range of mental health benefits, including improved concentration, memory and cognitive performance.

During sleep, the brain processes and consolidates the information acquired throughout the day, strengthening neural connections and facilitating the retention of memories. Lack of adequate sleep can impair the ability to concentrate, short-term memory and cognitive performance, negatively affecting daily functioning and learning ability.

In addition, sleep plays a key role in regulating emotions and emotional stability. During REM (rapid eye movement) sleep, there is intense brain activity involving the processing of emotions. Good quality sleep promotes proper emotional regulation, allowing emotions to be processed and integrated in a healthy way. On the other hand, sleep deprivation can lead to an emotional imbalance, increasing irritability, anxiety and emotional instability.

Adequate sleep also plays an important role in reducing stress and anxiety. During sleep, the body has the opportunity to recover from daily stress, allowing for physical and mental restoration. Lack of sleep can lead to an increased sensitivity to stress, hampering the ability to deal with emotional challenges and contributing to chronic anxiety.

Furthermore, sleep plays a role in preventing mental disorders such as depression and anxiety disorders. Chronic sleep deprivation has been linked to a higher risk of developing these disorders. On the other hand, a good quality of sleep is essential to promote mental health, prevent the onset of depressive symptoms and reduce the severity of anxiety disorders.

In summary, adequate sleep has a significant impact on mental health. It improves concentration, memory and cognitive performance, regulates emotions and promotes emotional stability, reduces stress and anxiety, and prevents the development of mental disorders such as depression and anxiety disorders. Prioritizing healthy sleep is essential to promoting mental health and emotional well-being.

## Influence of sleep on emotional abilities

Sleep plays a key role in emotional abilities, influencing the ability to deal with emotions, empathy and interpersonal relationships, as well as mood regulation and prevention of emotional swings.

A good quality of sleep is associated with a greater ability to deal with emotions in a healthy and effective way. During sleep, the brain has the opportunity to process and consolidate the day's emotional experiences, which allows for proper integration of emotions.

This results in greater emotional resilience, facilitating emotional regulation and the ability to deal with challenging situations.

Furthermore, adequate sleep is related to an improvement in empathy and interpersonal relationships. When we are well rested, we are better able to recognize and understand the emotions of others, showing greater empathy. This contributes to a better quality of interpersonal relationships, since empathy is essential for establishing healthy emotional connections and constructively resolving conflicts.

Mood regulation is another area influenced by sleep. During sleep, regulation of the neurochemical systems responsible for the balance of emotions occurs. A good quality of sleep contributes to proper mood regulation, helping to prevent excessive emotional swings, such as irritability, anger and sadness. On the other hand, chronic sleep deprivation can lead to emotional dysregulation, increasing susceptibility to sudden mood swings and hampering emotional stability.

In short, sleep plays a significant role in emotional abilities. It influences the ability to deal with emotions, improving emotional resilience and emotional regulation. Furthermore, adequate sleep promotes empathy and healthy interpersonal relationships, while preventing excessive emotional swings. Prioritizing healthy sleep is essential for developing and maintaining positive emotional skills, contributing to emotional and relational well-being.

*Statistics on sleep problems in today's society*

## Prevalence of sleep disorders

The prevalence of sleep disorders is a significant concern worldwide, affecting a large number of people. Several sleep disorders are common and have a significant impact on the quality of life and productivity of those affected.

Insomnia is one of the most prevalent sleep disorders. It is estimated that around 30% of the world's population suffers from insomnia at some point in their lives. Insomnia is characterized by difficulty falling asleep, staying asleep through the night, or waking up too early in the morning, resulting in insufficient, unrefreshing sleep. This lack of adequate sleep can have a significant impact on quality of life, causing daytime fatigue, difficulty concentrating, irritability and decreased cognitive performance.

Sleep apnea is also a common disorder, affecting approximately 5% of the adult population. Sleep apnea is characterized by pauses in breathing during sleep due to airway blockage. These breaks interrupt sleep and can lead to frequent awakenings throughout the night. Sleep apnea is associated with symptoms such as excessive daytime sleepiness, loud snoring, and difficulty concentrating. In addition, in the long term, sleep apnea can increase the risk of cardiovascular diseases such as hypertension and heart disease.

Another common sleep disorder is narcolepsy, which affects approximately 0.05% of the population. Narcolepsy is characterized by excessive daytime sleepiness, sudden bouts of overwhelming sleep, and sudden loss of muscle tone known as cataplexy. These symptoms can significantly interfere with daily life, causing difficulties in maintaining wakefulness, impairing academic and professional performance, and affecting social relationships.

In addition to these disorders, there are many others that affect sleep quality and overall health. This includes restless legs syndrome, bruxism (teeth grinding during sleep), sleepwalking, recurrent nightmares, and night terrors, among others. These disorders can have a significant impact on the quality of life and physical and mental health of those affected.

Sleep disorders have a wide-ranging impact on people's quality of life and productivity. Lack of adequate sleep negatively affects energy, concentration, mood and cognitive performance, interfering with work, studies, social activities and interpersonal relationships. Furthermore, chronic sleep deprivation is associated with a higher risk of developing chronic diseases such as heart disease, diabetes, obesity and mental disorders.

Sleep disorders are highly prevalent and have a significant impact on the quality of life and productivity of those affected. Awareness of these disorders is essential for seeking proper diagnosis and treatment in order to improve sleep quality, promote overall health, and maximize physical and mental well-being.

## Consequences of sleep deprivation

Sleep deprivation has a number of negative consequences for both physical and mental health. When we don't get enough quantity and quality of sleep, our bodies and minds are adversely impacted.

One of the most obvious effects of sleep deprivation is excessive daytime sleepiness, which can significantly increase the risk of accidents. Drowsiness affects the ability to concentrate, reaction time and decision-making, compromising safety at work, in traffic and in other daily activities. Chronic sleep deprivation is estimated to be associated with up to a three-fold increase in the risk of car accidents.

Furthermore, sleep deprivation is linked to a higher risk of developing chronic diseases such as diabetes and heart disease. Lack of adequate sleep negatively affects metabolism and the regulation of blood glucose levels, increasing insulin resistance and contributing to the development of type 2 diabetes.

Furthermore, sleep deprivation can lead to increased blood pressure, imbalance in cholesterol levels and alterations in the functioning of the cardiovascular system, increasing the risk of heart disease.

Sleep deprivation is also associated with a host of other negative physical and mental health consequences. It weakens the immune system, making the body more susceptible to infections and illnesses. A lack of adequate sleep compromises cell regeneration, impairs cognitive function, memory, concentration and academic and professional performance. In addition, sleep deprivation is linked to an increased risk of developing mental disorders such as depression, anxiety and general mental health problems.

Chronic sleep deprivation can also lead to changes in appetite and hormones related to weight regulation, contributing to weight gain and obesity. This occurs due to the imbalance of the hormones leptin and ghrelin, which regulate satiety and appetite. A lack of adequate sleep can also lead to changes in metabolism, favoring fat accumulation and increasing the risk of developing obesity.

Sleep deprivation has significant consequences for physical and mental health. It increases the risk of accidents due to drowsiness, is associated with the development of chronic diseases such as diabetes and heart disease, and has a negative impact on immune function, cognition, memory, mood and mental well-being. Prioritizing healthy sleep is essential to promoting overall health and maximizing proper body and mind functioning.

## Lifestyle and socioeconomic factors related to sleep

Various lifestyle and socioeconomic factors can have a significant impact on sleep quality. These factors can range from the use of technology and electronic devices to shift work and irregular hours, as well as stress, anxiety and everyday worries.

The influence of technology and electronic devices on sleep quality has become increasingly evident. Exposure to light emitted by smartphone, tablet, computer and television screens before bed can interfere with the circadian rhythm, suppress the production of melatonin (sleep hormone) and affect the quality of sleep. In addition, stimulating and emotionally engaging content from electronic devices can increase mental activity and make it difficult to transition into a relaxed state before bed. It is recommended to limit the use of electronic devices to at least one hour before bed to promote good sleep hygiene.

Shift work and irregular hours can also have a significant impact on your sleep routine. People who work night shifts, for example, often have difficulty synchronizing their circadian rhythm with their work schedule, resulting in chronic sleep deprivation. Additionally, irregular work schedules can lead to a lack of consistency in sleep schedules, making it difficult to establish a healthy routine. This can interfere with the quality and duration of sleep, negatively affecting health and well-being.

Stress, anxiety and daily worries are other factors that can interfere with adequate rest. Chronic stress can lead to a state of mental hyperactivity, making it difficult to transition into a relaxed state necessary for sleep. Anxiety and worries can lead to recurring, intrusive thoughts, making it difficult to turn your mind off before bed. These factors can result in difficulty falling asleep, frequent awakenings during the night, and unrefreshing sleep. Stress management strategies such as relaxation techniques, meditation practices, and cognitive-behavioral therapies can be helpful in promoting peaceful sleep.

It is important to recognize these lifestyle and socioeconomic factors that can interfere with sleep quality and seek ways to mitigate their negative effects. Setting limits on electronic device use before bed, maintaining a regular sleep routine even at irregular work hours, and developing effective strategies for managing stress and anxiety are all important steps to promoting healthy, restorative sleep.

*Purpose of Book: To provide information and strategies to help people sleep better*

<u>Importance of sleep education</u>

Sleep education plays a key role in promoting health and well-being. Awareness of the importance of sleep is essential for people to understand the benefits of adequate sleep and adopt healthy sleep practices. In addition, education empowers people to take care of their own sleep health, providing knowledge and strategies to improve the quality and quantity of sleep.

Awareness of the importance of sleep is essential because sleep is often neglected amid the demands of everyday life. Understanding that sleep is not a luxury, but a physiological necessity, helps people to prioritize adequate sleep time and conditions. Sleep education highlights the physical and mental benefits of good quality sleep, encouraging people to set aside enough time for sleep and adopt healthy sleep habits.

In addition, sleep education empowers people to take care of their own sleep health. By providing knowledge about the fundamentals of sleep, the factors that affect sleep quality and strategies to improve it, people become more aware of and responsible for their sleep-related choices. They learn to identify and avoid habits that impair sleep, such as excessive use of electronic devices before bed, and to implement practices that promote healthy sleep, such as creating an environment conducive to sleep and adopting regular bedtime routines. sleep.

By being empowered through sleep education, people can take active steps to improve their sleep quality. They become aware of the signs of insufficient sleep and the consequences of sleep deprivation, which motivates them to adopt positive changes in their daily routines to ensure adequate sleep. Education also helps people to identify possible sleep disorders and seek expert help when needed, thus improving their quality of life and overall health.

Sleep education plays an essential role in promoting sleep health. By making people aware of the importance of sleep for physical and mental well-being, and empowering them with knowledge and strategies to improve their sleep quality, education promotes a proactive approach to sleep. By becoming aware of and responsible for their own sleep health, people can adopt healthy sleep habits and reap the benefits of a well-rested life.

Sleep plays a crucial role in maintaining a healthy and balanced life, affecting not only physical health but mental, emotional and cognitive health as well. It needs to be emphasized that sleep is not an optional luxury, but a vital biological necessity.

During sleep, our body undergoes restoration, regeneration and repair processes. Adequate sleep strengthens the immune system, improving our ability to fight disease and infection.

It contributes to cardiovascular health by helping to regulate blood pressure, heart rate and blood vessel function. In addition, adequate sleep plays a key role in regulating weight and metabolism, influencing energy balance and regulating appetite-related hormones.

Regarding mental health, sleep plays an important role in memory consolidation and emotional processing. During sleep, our brain processes and stores information, which is crucial for learning and cognitive performance. In addition, adequate sleep helps regulate emotions, contributing to emotional stability, mental well-being and the ability to cope with stress and adversity.

By highlighting the importance of sleep as a fundamental pillar of health, I reaffirm my commitment to providing practical information and strategies to help you achieve quality sleep and a more balanced and healthy life. The main purpose of the book is to empower you to take active steps to improve your sleep health and enjoy the transformative benefits that adequate sleep can provide.

Throughout the book, information based on scientific evidence, proven practices and clear guidelines on how to establish a healthy sleep routine, improve the sleep environment, adopt relaxation techniques, deal with specific challenges and implement strategies for different stages of life will be presented. . The book provides a comprehensive set of tools and resources to help you identify your sleep problems, understand their causes, and implement positive changes in your lives.

Through this commitment, the book aims to promote a more balanced, healthy and fulfilling life, recognizing that adequate sleep is one of the main pillars to achieve this goal.

# Fundamentals of Sleep

*The science behind sleep: the circadian cycle, sleep stages and their characteristics*

<u>the circadian cycle</u>

The circadian cycle is a biological rhythm that regulates sleep and wake patterns over approximately 24 hours. It plays a crucial role in regulating sleep and balancing our body. This cycle is mainly influenced by light and dark.

During the day, exposure to light, especially natural light, has a significant impact on the circadian cycle. Sunlight helps suppress the production of the sleep hormone melatonin and keeps our brains alert and awake. This is why exposure to light during the day is beneficial in keeping us awake, alert and energized.

As night falls and the light diminishes, our bodies begin to produce melatonin, the sleep hormone. Darkness stimulates the release of this hormone, signaling to our body that it is time to relax and sleep. On the other hand, exposure to light, especially the blue light emitted by electronic devices, can disrupt melatonin production and make falling asleep more difficult.

Therefore, it is essential to create an environment conducive to sleep at night. Reducing exposure to bright light before bed, including light emitted from electronic devices, can help make it easier to fall asleep. In addition, creating a dark and quiet environment in the bedroom, blocking excessive light and maintaining a pleasant temperature, contributes to the quality of sleep.

Understanding the role of the circadian cycle in sleep regulation and the influence of light and dark is key to promoting healthy sleep. By adopting habits that respect this cycle, we can improve our ability to fall asleep and wake up at the right time, providing quality sleep.

So remember to take care of your exposure to light by taking advantage of natural light during the day and reducing exposure to bright light before bed. Creating a sleep-friendly environment that is dark, quiet, and comfortable also contributes to adequate rest. Respecting the circadian cycle and adopting these practices helps promote healthy and restorative sleep.

## sleep stages

Sleep is composed of different stages, each with specific characteristics and brain activities. These stages are divided into REM (rapid eye movement) sleep and non-REM sleep, and switching between them plays a key role in healthy, restorative sleep.

During non-REM sleep, our body goes through three stages: light sleep, deep sleep and slow wave sleep. At the onset of sleep, we enter the light sleep stage, in which we are still in a transitional state between wakefulness and sleep. Light sleep is characterized by slower brain activity and greater sensitivity to external stimuli. As sleep progresses, we enter the deep sleep stage, also known as slow wave sleep. At this stage, brain activity slows down even more and the body recovers from physical and mental fatigue. It is during deep sleep that processes of restoration and regeneration of the organism occur.

In contrast, REM sleep is a stage characterized by a pattern of rapid eye movements and an increase in brain activity. At this stage, we dream more often and our muscles are relaxed, almost paralyzed. REM sleep plays an important role in memory consolidation and emotional processing. Furthermore, this stage is believed to be related to creativity, problem solving, and cognitive development.

Alternating between REM and non-REM stages throughout the night is essential for healthy, restorative sleep. This alternation is known as the sleep cycle. During the first half of the night, most sleep is comprised of non-REM stages, with deep sleep predominating. As the night progresses, periods of REM sleep become longer and more frequent. This sequence of REM and non-REM stages is important for a number of physiological and mental functions.

A healthy sleep cycle, with proper alternation between REM and non-REM stages, allows our bodies to recover, repair tissues, consolidate memories and regulate emotions. Deviations in this alternation, such as unbalanced sleep or lack of REM sleep, can lead to health and well-being problems, such as fatigue, difficulty concentrating, mood swings and even cognitive impairment.

Therefore, it is essential to value all stages of sleep, both REM and non-REM, and seek an adequate balance between them. Good sleep hygiene, an environment conducive to rest and the adoption of healthy sleep practices can contribute to an adequate alternation between these stages and promote quality sleep that is restorative and revitalizing.

## Functions and benefits of sleep

Sleep performs a variety of vital functions for our body and mind, with benefits that go beyond just resting.

One of the most fascinating aspects of sleep is its role in memory consolidation and learning. During sleep, our brain processes and stores information acquired throughout the day, strengthening neural connections and improving information retention. Studies show that a good night's sleep after learning is associated with better performance on tests of memory and learning.

Furthermore, sleep plays a crucial role in cell repair and regeneration. During sleep, the body releases hormones that promote growth and repair of damaged tissue. This includes the production of proteins that aid in wound healing, muscle recovery and new cell synthesis. It is during sleep that repair of damage caused by stress, daily activities and exposure to toxins occurs.

Another important function of sleep is hormonal balance and appetite regulation.

During sleep, hormonal changes occur that affect appetite and metabolism. Lack of sleep is associated with elevated levels of the hormone ghrelin, which stimulates appetite, and reduced levels of the hormone leptin, which signals feelings of fullness. This hormonal dysfunction can lead to increased appetite, cravings for high-calorie foods, and difficulty maintaining a healthy weight.

Additionally, sleep plays a crucial role in cardiovascular, immune, and metabolic health. During sleep, processes occur that help regulate blood pressure, immune system function, and carbohydrate metabolism. Sleep deprivation is associated with a higher risk of developing cardiovascular disease, impaired immune system and changes in metabolism, including insulin resistance and increased risk of obesity and type 2 diabetes.

These are just a few examples of the functions and benefits of sleep for our body and mind. Adequate sleep plays a key role in our overall health and well-being. Therefore, it is essential to value and prioritize sleep, adopting healthy sleep habits and creating an environment conducive to quality rest. In this way, we can take advantage of all the benefits that sleep provides, promoting a healthier and more balanced life.

## *Optimal sleep duration for different age groups*

### Sleep recommendations by age group

Sleep recommendations vary by age group, as sleep needs evolve as we grow. Let's take a deeper look at sleep recommendations by age group:

**Infants and young children (0 to 3 years):** During the first few years of life, babies and toddlers have varying sleep needs, depending on their age. Generally, newborns need about 14 to 17 hours of sleep a day, while older babies (3 to 12 months) need approximately 12 to 15 hours of sleep. As children approach 2 to 3 years of age, their need for sleep decreases a bit, to around 11 to 14 hours a day.

**School age children (4 to 12 years old):** In this age group, the general recommendation is that children sleep 9 to 12 hours a night. Adequate sleep is essential for growth, cognitive development and good school performance. Establishing a consistent sleep routine, with regular sleep and wake times, can be especially beneficial for children in this age group.

**Teenagers (13 to 18 years old):** During adolescence, sleep needs are still high. It is recommended that teenagers sleep 8 to 10 hours a night. However, many teenagers struggle to get enough sleep due to biological changes, academic and social pressures. It is important to promote an environment conducive to sleep, limit the use of electronic devices before bed, and encourage a regular sleep routine.

**Adults (18 to 64 years):** For adults, the recommendation is 7 to 9 hours of sleep per night. However, it is worth noting that individual needs may vary. Some people may feel refreshed on less sleep, while others need more to feel rested. The important thing is to find the amount of sleep that allows you to function properly during the day, maintaining a healthy balance between work, life and rest.

**Seniors (over 65 years old):** As we age, sleep needs may decrease a bit. The recommendation for seniors is 7 to 8 hours of sleep per night. However, as with adults, individual needs can vary. It is important to respect changes in sleep patterns that may occur with age, such as shorter periods of sleep or night awakenings, and seek to create an environment conducive to quality sleep.

These are general sleep recommendations by age group, but remember that everyone is unique and may have individual sleep needs. It's important to pay attention to your own body's signals and adjust your sleep routine accordingly to what brings you adequate rest and revitalization. Prioritizing sleep and adopting healthy sleep hygiene practices at all ages is essential to promoting a balanced and healthy life.

## Importance of individuality

It is crucial to recognize and value individuality when it comes to sleep needs. While there are general sleep recommendations by age group, it's important to understand that individual sleep needs can vary considerably from person to person.

Several factors can influence individual sleep needs. One of these factors is genetics. Studies have shown that optimal sleep duration may have a genetic basis. Some people may feel refreshed and alert with less sleep, while others need more hours to feel rested. These genetic differences can influence how much sleep a person needs to function optimally.

In addition, activity levels can also affect individual sleep needs. People with more active lifestyles or those who engage in intense physical activities may have a greater demand for sleep to recover properly. The physical and mental effort exerted during the day can increase the need for rest and restful sleep during the night.

Other individual factors such as health status, stress level, cognitive and emotional demands can also influence a person's sleep needs. For example, someone who is going through a period of intense stress may need more sleep to help with emotional and physical recovery.

It's important to respect and honor these individual differences when it comes to sleep. It's critical to listen to your own body's signals, be mindful of sleep quality, and adjust your sleep routine according to what works best for you.

So don't compare yourself to others regarding sleep. Recognize that your individual needs may be different and make adjustments according to what brings you a sense of rest and well-being. Individuality in sleep is an essential part of achieving healthy sleep and a balanced life.

*Impact of inadequate sleep on health and well-being*

## Consequences of sleep deprivation

Sleep deprivation can have a number of negative consequences for our health and well-being. Let's explore these consequences in more detail:

**Fatigue and daytime sleepiness:** Sleep deprivation leads to a constant feeling of tiredness and drowsiness during the day. Lack of adequate rest prevents our body and mind from rejuvenating, resulting in low energy and lack of willingness to carry out daily activities.

**Difficulties with concentration, memory and cognitive performance:** A night of insufficient sleep can negatively affect our cognitive abilities. Lack of sleep compromises the ability to concentrate, impairs memory and makes learning difficult. Tasks that require attention and focus become more challenging.

**Increased risk of accidents and decreased ability to make decisions:** Drowsiness resulting from sleep deprivation can compromise our ability to react and make decisions. This increases the risk of traffic accidents, accidents at work and other incidents in activities that require alertness and coordination.

**Mood swings, irritability, and decreased ability to handle stress:** Sleep deprivation has a significant impact on our emotional state. When we are sleep deprived, we tend to be more irritable, impatient and emotionally unstable. In addition, our ability to handle stress decreases, which can lead to relationship problems and decreased psychological well-being.

**Negative impact on physical health:** Lack of adequate sleep is associated with a higher risk of developing chronic diseases. Chronic sleep deprivation can lead to high blood pressure, an increased risk of cardiovascular diseases such as heart disease and stroke, and an increased likelihood of developing type 2 diabetes and obesity. This is due to hormonal imbalances such as decreased insulin sensitivity and changes in carbohydrate and fat metabolism.

These are just some of the consequences of sleep deprivation. It is critical to recognize the importance of adequate sleep for our physical and mental health. Prioritizing sleep and adopting healthy sleep hygiene practices are essential steps to prevent these negative consequences and promote a balanced and healthy life.

## Relationship between sleep and mental health

The relationship between sleep and mental health is deep and complex. Inadequate sleep can play a significant role in the development and worsening of mental disorders such as depression and anxiety. Likewise, mental health issues can negatively affect sleep, creating a vicious cycle where one intensifies the other.

Lack of adequate sleep can contribute to the emergence of mental disorders. Studies have shown a close link between sleep deprivation and depression. Lack of sleep can affect mood, increase emotional sensitivity and reduce the ability to cope with stress, factors that can contribute to the development of depression. In addition, sleep deprivation interferes with chemical and neural processes in the brain related to mood and emotions, which can trigger or exacerbate depressive symptoms.

Likewise, the relationship between inadequate sleep and anxiety is equally significant. Sleep deprivation negatively affects anxiety levels, increasing feelings of tension, worry and irritability. Furthermore, anxiety can lead to difficulties falling asleep and maintaining quality sleep, creating a cycle where lack of sleep intensifies anxiety symptoms, and anxiety, in turn, negatively affects sleep.

This vicious cycle between sleep problems and mental health can become harmful. Lack of adequate sleep can lead to an increased risk of developing mental disorders, as well as worsening symptoms in people who already have a diagnosis. On the other hand, the presence of mental disorders, such as depression and anxiety, can interfere with the quality and quantity of sleep, making it more difficult to fall asleep, stay asleep or have restful sleep.

It is critical to address both sleep problems and mental disorders in an integrated way. Treating mental health and promoting adequate sleep are interconnected aspects. Therapeutic approaches such as cognitive behavioral therapy for insomnia can be effective in treating both. In addition, adopting healthy sleep hygiene practices and seeking strategies to manage stress and anxiety can contribute to improving sleep quality and overall mental health.

Therefore, it is important to recognize the bidirectional relationship between sleep and mental health. Taking care of adequate sleep is an essential aspect of promoting mental health and emotional well-being. Likewise, addressing mental health issues can also have a positive impact on sleep quality. Prioritizing both sleep and mental health is key to breaking the vicious cycle and promoting a balanced and healthy life.

## Importance of quality sleep for overall well-being

Quality sleep plays a key role in our overall well-being. Let's explore some of the ways in which adequate sleep positively affects our vitality, quality of life and overall health.

Promotion of vitality, energy and productivity: Adequate quality sleep gives us the vitality and energy needed to face the day. When we sleep well, we wake up refreshed and ready to tackle daily activities with more energy and focus. Adequate sleep is also linked to better cognitive performance, improved memory, concentration and decision-making.

This allows us to be more productive and efficient in our daily tasks.

Improved quality of life and interpersonal relationships: Quality sleep is directly linked to our quality of life. When we sleep well, we experience a general sense of well-being and contentment. Adequate sleep helps us regulate our emotions, which allows us to better handle stress and have healthier relationships. In addition, quality sleep also contributes to mental health, reducing the risk of developing mental disorders such as depression and anxiety.

Immune System Strengthening and Disease Prevention: Adequate sleep plays an important role in maintaining a healthy immune system. During sleep, our body produces and releases cytokines, substances that are essential for proper immune response. Sleep deprivation is associated with a decrease in the production of these substances, which can compromise immune function and increase the risk of infectious diseases. Therefore, adequate quality sleep is essential to strengthen the immune system and prevent illness.

In addition to these benefits, adequate sleep is also associated with a host of other positive health aspects, such as hormone regulation, maintaining a healthy weight, cardiovascular health, and the prevention of chronic diseases such as diabetes and heart disease.

It is important to prioritize quality sleep in our daily routine. Adopting healthy sleep hygiene practices, such as having a regular sleep routine, creating an environment conducive to rest and adopting relaxation strategies before bed, are important steps to promote quality sleep. By taking care of our sleep, we are investing in our overall well-being and enjoying a more balanced, healthy and fulfilling life.

***

It is essential to understand the science of sleep in order to optimize its quality and duration, and thus promote a healthier and more balanced life. By understanding the mechanisms and benefits of sleep, we can take concrete steps to improve our sleep routine and maximize its positive effects on our health and well-being.

Sleep deprivation can have significant negative consequences on our physical and mental health. Lack of adequate sleep is associated with a host of health problems, such as an increased risk of cardiovascular disease, diabetes, obesity, impaired immune system and shorter life expectancy. In addition, sleep deprivation affects our mental health, contributing to increased anxiety, depression, irritability and difficulty concentrating.

Furthermore, it is important to highlight that adequate sleep is not just a luxury, but a fundamental necessity for our health and well-being. When we get enough sleep, we feel more energetic, alert, emotionally balanced and able to deal with everyday challenges. Quality sleep allows us to be more productive, creative and efficient in our daily activities.

# Identifying Sleep Disorders

*Main sleep disorders: insomnia, sleep apnea, narcolepsy, restless legs syndrome, among others*

<u>Insomnia</u>

Insomnia is a common sleep disorder that affects many people across the world. It is characterized by persistent difficulty falling asleep or staying asleep through the night, even when there is an adequate opportunity to sleep. Insomnia can be a temporary problem, lasting a few days or weeks, or it can become chronic, persisting for an extended period.

There are different types of insomnia, each with its own distinct characteristics. Sleep reconciliation insomnia is characterized by difficulties falling asleep early in the night, while sleep maintenance insomnia involves frequent awakenings during the night, with difficulty returning to sleep. In addition, insomnia can be classified as acute (short-term) or chronic (long-term) depending on the duration of symptoms.

Several risk factors are associated with insomnia. Stress is one of the main triggers for insomnia, as worry and anxiety can interfere with falling asleep and sleeping at night. Anxiety and depression are also commonly associated with insomnia, forming a negative cycle in which insomnia can exacerbate symptoms of anxiety and depression, and vice versa. In addition, certain medical conditions such as chronic pain, respiratory illnesses, hormonal disorders and neurological diseases can contribute to the occurrence of insomnia.

Other risk factors include the use of certain medications, excessive consumption of caffeine or alcohol, an unfavorable sleep environment such as inappropriate noise and temperature, and irregular sleep habits. Lifestyle factors such as irregular work schedules and excessive use of electronic devices before bed can also play a role in the occurrence of insomnia.

It is important to address insomnia comprehensively, identifying underlying causes and implementing effective strategies to improve sleep. This may involve adopting healthy sleep hygiene practices, such as establishing a regular sleep routine, creating an environment conducive to rest, limiting exposure to stimulating stimuli before bed, and looking for ways to manage stress and anxiety. In some cases, the intervention of health professionals such as doctors and sleep therapists may be necessary for proper treatment of insomnia.

By understanding the different types of insomnia, the associated risk factors, and the strategies available to manage it, affected individuals can take steps to improve the quality of their sleep and consequently their health and well-being. The approach to insomnia must be personalized, taking into account individual circumstances and needs, to promote restorative sleep and a balanced life.

## Sleep apnea

Sleep apnea is a sleep disorder characterized by repeated episodes of interrupted breathing during sleep. During these episodes, breathing temporarily stops due to the collapse of the upper airways, resulting in a decrease in blood oxygen levels. These breathing pauses can last a few seconds to minutes and occur several times throughout the night.

One of the most common symptoms of sleep apnea is loud, persistent snoring while sleeping. Snoring occurs due to limited air passage through narrowed airways. In addition, breathing pauses during sleep can lead to brief and fragmented awakenings, interrupting the normal sleep cycle. As a result, people with sleep apnea often experience excessive daytime sleepiness, fatigue, lack of energy, and difficulty maintaining focus and concentration during the day.

Several risk factors are associated with sleep apnea. Obesity is one of the main factors, since excess adipose tissue in the neck region can compress the airways, making it difficult for air to pass through. Advanced age also increases the risk of sleep apnea, as airway tissues tend to lose elasticity and support over the years. In addition, family history of sleep apnea, presence of diseases such as diabetes, hypertension and cardiovascular disease, smoking and use of alcohol and sedatives are also factors that increase the risk of developing sleep apnea.

Sleep apnea is a condition that deserves proper attention and treatment, as it can have negative consequences for health and well-being. Chronic oxygen deprivation due to repeated breathing pauses can lead to serious health problems such as high blood pressure, cardiovascular disease, stroke, type 2 diabetes and cognitive problems.

If you suspect you are suffering from sleep apnea, it is critical to seek proper medical evaluation and treatment. Diagnosis usually involves conducting a sleep study, which monitors various body functions during sleep to detect the presence of breathing disorders. Treatment may involve lifestyle changes, such as losing weight, avoiding alcohol and sedatives, and sleeping in a proper position. In more severe cases, it may be necessary to use devices such as CPAP (continuous positive airway pressure) or even surgery to correct physical obstructions in the airways.

Awareness of sleep apnea symptoms, risk factors and treatment options is essential to help people seek medical help and improve their sleep quality and overall health. With proper treatment, it is possible to control the symptoms of sleep apnea, improve sleep quality and reduce the risk of complications associated with the disease.

## narcolepsy

Narcolepsy is a chronic neurological disorder that affects sleep and wakefulness. It is characterized by excessive and overwhelming sleepiness during the day, resulting in uncontrollable sleep attacks, in which the person may fall asleep suddenly and in inappropriate situations, such as while talking, driving or working. These sleep attacks can last from a few seconds to minutes.

In addition to excessive daytime sleepiness, narcolepsy has other distinct symptoms. Cataplexy is one of the most characteristic symptoms and consists of the sudden and temporary loss of muscle control in response to strong emotions such as surprise, laughter or anger. During an episode of cataplexy, the muscles can become weak or even temporarily paralyzed, causing the person to fall. Other common symptoms include sleep hallucinations, which are vivid, vivid experiences that occur when falling asleep or waking up, and sleep paralysis, which is the temporary inability to move or speak when falling asleep or waking up.

The exact causes of narcolepsy are still not completely understood, but it is believed that there is a complex interaction of genetic and environmental factors. Studies have shown a significant association between narcolepsy and a genetic predisposition, indicating that certain genes may be involved in the development of the disease. Additionally, narcolepsy is associated with dysfunction of the neurotransmitter hypocretin (also known as orexin), which plays an important role in regulating sleep and wakefulness. In narcolepsy, there is a decrease in the production of hypocretin or a failure to transmit signals related to this neurotransmitter.

Narcolepsy can have a significant impact on the lives of those affected, interfering with their daily activities and quality of life. Excessive daytime sleepiness can negatively affect academic and professional performance, as well as social relationships and safety, especially in situations that require attention and vigilance, such as driving. Cataplexy and sleep hallucinations can also be a source of embarrassment and limitations in daily activities.

While there is no cure for narcolepsy, treatment is aimed at controlling symptoms and improving the quality of life for those affected. This usually involves combining medications such as stimulants to combat daytime drowsiness and antidepressants to manage cataplexy and associated emotional symptoms. In addition, it is important to adopt sleep management strategies, such as establishing regular sleep routines, taking planned naps during the day, and creating a suitable sleeping environment.

Awareness of narcolepsy is critical to ensuring proper diagnosis and treatment. Understanding the symptoms, possible causes, and treatment options can help those affected seek medical help and find ways to manage their symptoms. With proper treatment and support, it is possible to control the symptoms of narcolepsy and lead a full and productive life.

## Restless legs syndrome (RLS)

Restless legs syndrome (RLS) is a neurological condition that manifests itself as an uncomfortable feeling in the legs and an overwhelming urge to move them. These symptoms usually occur during periods of rest or relaxation, such as at night when the person is lying in bed. The unpleasant sensation in the legs is described as a tingling, crawling, itching, burning, or "crawling" sensation. These sensations can vary in intensity and can be relieved temporarily by moving the legs.

RLS symptoms can cause significant discomfort and interfere with the ability to fall asleep and stay asleep, resulting in daytime sleepiness, fatigue, and irritability. In addition, RLS can negatively affect quality of life, as affected people may experience difficulties in daily activities and interpersonal relationships due to the need to move their legs to relieve symptoms.

Although the exact cause of RLS is not fully understood, several factors are thought to contribute to its development. Iron deficiency is one of the known causes of RLS, and iron supplementation can help alleviate symptoms in some people. In addition, RLS may be associated with neurological diseases such as Parkinson's disease and peripheral neuropathies. The use of certain medications, such as antidepressants, antihistamines, and motion sickness medications, can also trigger or worsen RLS symptoms in some people.

The diagnosis of RLS is based on the patient's reported symptoms and a clinical assessment. There are no specific tests to diagnose RLS, but in some cases laboratory tests may be ordered to assess iron levels and rule out other underlying causes.

Treatment of RLS is aimed at relieving symptoms and improving quality of life. This may involve identifying and treating underlying conditions such as iron deficiency. In addition, medications may be prescribed to help control symptoms, such as dopamine agonists, opioids, or antiseizure medications. In addition, adopting healthy sleep hygiene measures, such as establishing regular sleep routines, avoiding stimulants before bed, and creating an adequate environment for rest, can help minimize RLS symptoms.

Awareness of RLS is important to ensure proper diagnosis and treatment. Understanding the symptoms, contributing factors, and available treatment options can help those affected seek medical help and find ways to manage their symptoms. With proper treatment, many people are able to control RLS symptoms and enjoy a better quality of life.

## When to seek specialist medical help

### Recognizing the need for professional assistance

Recognizing the need for professional assistance when a sleep disorder is suspected is extremely important to ensure an accurate assessment and initiation of appropriate treatment. There are certain indicators that can signal the presence of a sleep disorder and justify seeking medical help.

The persistence of symptoms is one of the main indicators that a sleep disorder may be present. If you experience sleep-related symptoms, such as difficulty falling asleep, waking up frequently during the night, loud snoring, excessive daytime sleepiness, or uncomfortable sensations in your legs, and these symptoms persist for an extended period of time, it is important to seek medical evaluation. Symptoms that consistently interfere with sleep quality and negatively affect your daily life are signs that there may be an underlying sleep disorder.

Significant impact on quality of life is another indicator that professional assistance is needed. If sleep symptoms affect your daily activities, job performance, relationships, or emotional well-being, it is critical to seek medical evaluation. Sleep disturbances can have a profound impact on quality of life, causing chronic fatigue, concentration difficulties, mood swings and long-term health problems. So if you find that your symptoms are interfering with your overall functioning and well-being, it's important to seek help.

Seeking medical evaluation to get an accurate diagnosis and start proper treatment is key to dealing with sleep disorders. A doctor who specializes in sleep disorders will be able to perform a detailed assessment of your symptoms, medical history and sleep patterns. This may involve performing specific tests, such as a sleep study or laboratory tests, to aid in the diagnosis. An accurate diagnosis is crucial to determine the most appropriate treatment for you.

In addition, professional assistance will allow you to obtain personalized guidance and receive adequate recommendations to improve the quality of your sleep. Treatments for sleep disorders can vary widely, from lifestyle changes and behavioral therapies to the use of medical devices or medications, depending on the specific disorder. A specialist doctor will be able to advise you on the best treatment options based on your individual needs.

Seeking medical help is a positive step towards taking care of your health and well-being. Don't hesitate to seek professional evaluation if you suspect a sleep disorder. Proper diagnosis and timely treatment can make a significant difference to your quality of life by promoting healthy, revitalizing sleep.

## Health professionals specializing in sleep disorders

The diagnosis and treatment of sleep disorders involve a multidisciplinary team of specialized health professionals. Several medical specialties play important roles in the diagnosis, treatment and management of sleep disorders, ensuring a comprehensive and personalized approach for each patient.

Sleep medicine specialists are highly trained professionals who focus specifically on sleep disorders. They have in-depth knowledge about different sleep disorders, their causes, symptoms, diagnosis and treatment. These specialists are trained to perform detailed clinical assessments, interpret sleep study results, and prescribe appropriate treatments. They may be physicians with a background in sleep medicine or pulmonologists with expertise in this field.

Pulmonologists are doctors who specialize in the diagnosis and treatment of lung conditions, including sleep-related breathing disorders such as sleep apnea. They are uniquely qualified to assess lung function, identify upper airway obstructions and prescribe specific treatments such as continuous positive airway pressure (CPAP) devices for the treatment of sleep apnea.

Neurologists are doctors who specialize in the diagnosis and treatment of disorders of the nervous system, including sleep-related neurological disorders such as narcolepsy. They are familiar with the neurological changes that can occur during sleep and are trained to identify and treat sleep disorders of neurological origin. In addition, neurologists can also treat other sleep-related conditions, such as movement disorders during sleep.

Psychiatrists are doctors who specialize in the diagnosis and treatment of mental disorders. Although they are not specifically specialized in sleep medicine, they play a key role in the management of sleep disorders, especially when there is a close relationship between sleep disorders and mental disorders, such as insomnia associated with anxiety or depression. Psychiatrists can assess and treat underlying mental disorders that may be contributing to sleep disturbances, as well as prescribe appropriate medications to treat these conditions.

Together, these healthcare professionals who specialize in sleep disorders collaborate to provide an integrated, holistic approach to the diagnosis, treatment, and management of sleep disorders. They work closely together, sharing information and experiences to ensure that each patient receives the most appropriate and personalized care. When seeking professional help for a sleep disorder, it is important to see the right doctor for the specific type of sleep disorder you are experiencing. They will be able to carry out a comprehensive assessment and provide you with the appropriate treatment to improve your sleep quality and overall well-being.

## Available treatments and therapies

There are a variety of treatments and therapies available to help manage and treat sleep disorders. These options span medical approaches, behavioral therapies, and lifestyle changes, providing a comprehensive approach to meeting each person's individual needs.

Medical approaches are often used in the treatment of sleep disorders. Medications may be prescribed to help improve symptoms and promote more regular, restorative sleep. Sleep medications include sedatives, hypnotics, and other agents that can help induce sleep. However, it is important to emphasize that the use of medications must be done under proper medical supervision, as some may have side effects and associated risks.

Continuous positive airway pressure (CPAP) therapy is a common approach to treating sleep apnea. This device consists of a mask that is worn during sleep to provide a constant flow of air, helping to keep the airway open and preventing airway obstruction. CPAP is highly effective in treating sleep apnea, reducing symptoms and improving sleep quality.

Oral devices can also be used to treat sleep disorders such as sleep apnea. These devices are designed to position the jaw and tongue to keep the airway open during sleep. They can be especially helpful for people who have mild to moderate sleep apnea or who cannot tolerate CPAP use.

Behavioral therapies are an important approach in the treatment of sleep disorders. Cognitive behavioral therapy for insomnia (CBT-I) is an effective therapy that aims to identify and modify the thought and behavior patterns that contribute to insomnia. CBT-I includes relaxation techniques, sleep hygiene, stress management strategies and behavioral adjustments that help improve sleep quality in a natural and lasting way.

Additionally, relaxation techniques such as breathing exercises, meditation, and yoga can be beneficial in treating sleep disorders. These practices help calm the mind, reduce stress, and promote a state of relaxation that makes it easier to fall asleep. Practicing relaxation techniques regularly can help improve sleep quality and promote a general sense of well-being.

In addition to medical and therapeutic approaches, lifestyle changes play a key role in the treatment of sleep disorders. This includes establishing a regular sleep routine, creating an environment conducive to rest, avoiding stimulants such as caffeine and nicotine before bed, and adopting self-care practices such as regular exercise and a balanced diet. These lifestyle changes are essential for promoting healthy sleep and improving sleep quality in the long term.

*\*\**

Recognizing the signs of possible sleep disorders is essential to ensure an adequate approach and adequate treatment. There are some common signs that may indicate the presence of a sleep disorder, such as persistent difficulty falling asleep, frequent waking during the night, excessive sleepiness during the day, loud snoring, and uncomfortable sensations in the legs. If you experience these symptoms on a regular basis and they are interfering with your sleep quality and general well-being, it is important to consider seeking specialist medical help.

By seeking expert medical help, you will be able to get a proper diagnosis and a personalized treatment plan. A healthcare professional who specializes in sleep disorders will be able to assess your symptoms, medical history and sleep patterns to identify the underlying cause of the problem. This may involve conducting a sleep study, laboratory tests and a detailed clinical evaluation. Based on this assessment, the professional will be able to provide an accurate diagnosis and recommend the most appropriate treatment for your specific case.

It is essential to highlight the variety of treatment options available to improve sleep quality and general well-being. There are medical approaches such as the use of specific medications, continuous positive airway pressure (CPAP) therapy for sleep apnea, and oral devices for sleep-related breathing disorders. Behavioral therapies such as Cognitive Behavioral Therapy for Insomnia (CBT-I) are also effective in treating sleep disorders as they address the behavioral and cognitive factors that contribute to insomnia. Additionally, lifestyle changes such as adopting a consistent sleep routine, creating an environment conducive to sleep, and practicing relaxation techniques can have a significant impact on sleep quality.

Each person is unique and may respond differently to different treatments, so it's important to seek professional guidance to find the approach that best suits your individual needs.

Adequate sleep plays a key role in overall health and well-being. Don't hesitate to seek medical help if you suspect a sleep disorder. A proper diagnosis and a personalized treatment plan can make a significant difference in your quality of life, helping you to achieve restful sleep and a more balanced and healthy life.

## Hygiene do Sono

*Establishing a healthy sleep routine: regular schedules, suitable environment, relaxing rituals*

## regular hours

Keeping regular sleep schedules, waking up and going to bed every day, is essential to promote quality sleep and ensure the proper functioning of our circadian rhythm. The circadian rhythm is the approximately 24-hour biological cycle that regulates our sleep and wake patterns. It is influenced by factors such as exposure to light and dark, and plays a crucial role in regulating our physiological and behavioral processes.

When we follow a regular sleep pattern, we synchronize our circadian rhythm, allowing it to naturally adjust to changes in light and dark throughout the day. This strengthens our internal clock, helping us fall asleep more easily, get deeper sleep, and wake up naturally and refreshed in the morning. Conversely, having irregular sleep schedules, such as sleeping late and waking up late on weekends, can lead to circadian rhythm dysregulation and cause difficulties falling asleep and waking up during the week.

Establishing regular sleep schedules is especially important because our bodies function best when they follow a consistent schedule. By adopting a consistent sleep routine, our body learns to prepare for sleep and wake up at certain times. This means that our physiological and hormonal systems are primed to optimize sleep when bedtime comes and to wake us up more easily in the morning.

Following regular sleep schedules also benefits other aspects of our daily lives. When we have a consistent schedule, our daily routine becomes more predictable, which helps us plan our activities and appointments more efficiently. In addition, establishing regular sleep schedules helps us to balance our other daily habits, such as food, exercise and time to relax. This regularity contributes to a more balanced and healthy lifestyle.

However, it's important to point out that establishing regular sleep schedules doesn't mean we should be inflexible all the time. It is normal for occasional variations to occur, such as in special situations or travel. The important thing is to maintain regularity as much as possible and resume your regular routine as soon as possible.

To establish regular sleep schedules, it is recommended to set a consistent bedtime and wake-up time, including on weekends. It's important to consider the amount of sleep you need and adjust your schedules accordingly. Gradually, your body will adapt to this routine and begin to naturally feel sleepy and more alert at your desired times.

In short, maintaining regular sleep schedules is key to synchronizing your circadian rhythm and promoting quality sleep. This consistency helps our body adjust to the natural cycle of light and dark, providing a better quality of sleep and a more refreshing awakening. By adopting regular sleep schedules, you will be investing in your overall health and well-being, contributing to a balanced and healthy life.

## suitable environment

Creating a suitable sleeping environment is essential to promoting restful, restful sleep. A cool, dark and quiet bedroom can make all the difference in the quality of your sleep and your overall well-being.

One of the main considerations when creating an environment conducive to sleep is the temperature of the room. The ideal temperature may vary from person to person, but in general, a cool, slightly cooler environment is preferable. The ideal temperature is usually around 18 to 20 degrees Celsius. It's important to adjust your bedroom temperature to your personal preferences and make sure you're comfortable sleeping. Good ventilation, the use of fans or air conditioning can help regulate the temperature of the room.

Darkness is an important factor in promoting adequate sleep. Exposure to light before bed can suppress the production of melatonin, a hormone that helps regulate sleep. Therefore, it is recommended to create a dark environment in the bedroom. Use blackout curtains or blinds to block outside light, especially at night. If there are unwanted lights in the room, such as street lights or electronics, you may want to consider using sleep shades or window plugs to block out unwanted light.

Silence is another important factor in ensuring peaceful sleep. External noises such as traffic, noisy neighbors or even a partner's snoring can disturb sleep and interfere with its quality. To minimize external noise, you can use earplugs, white noise machines, or even headphones with relaxing music or calming natural sounds. These techniques help mask unwanted sounds and create a more peaceful sleep environment.

Choosing a suitable mattress and pillows also plays a key role in creating a conducive sleeping environment. Preferences for mattresses and pillows can vary from person to person, as everyone has individual needs for support and comfort. It's important to choose a mattress and pillow that provide the level of support you need for your posture and personal preferences. Experimenting with different types of mattresses and pillows, such as memory foam, latex, or spring, can help you find the best fit for you.

When creating a suitable sleeping environment, take into account all these aspects: temperature, darkness, silence and the comfort of the mattress and pillows. Customize your environment to your individual preferences and make adjustments as needed to ensure restful, restful sleep. Creating an environment conducive to sleep is an important part of sleep care and can have a significant impact on the quality of your night's rest and your overall well-being.

### relaxing rituals

Incorporating relaxing rituals before bed can be an effective strategy to prepare the body and mind for restful sleep. These rituals help signal the brain that it's time to relax and prepare for the night's rest. By adopting a consistent routine of relaxing rituals, you can create an environment conducive to sleep and promote a smooth transition from wakefulness to sleep.

There are several relaxing ritual practices that you can try before bed. Taking a warm bath or relaxing bath can be an effective way to relax your muscles and relieve tension in your body. Warm water has a calming effect and can help induce a feeling of relaxation and drowsiness. Additionally, reading a book or engaging in quiet activities, such as listening to soft music, can help calm the mind and prepare it for sleep. Avoid, however, reading or activities that might stimulate your mind or cause you to be preoccupied, as this can interfere with your ability to relax and fall asleep.

It is important to avoid using electronic devices, such as smartphones, tablets and computers, before going to bed. The light emitted by these devices, especially blue light, can interfere with the production of melatonin, the sleep hormone. Using electronic devices before bed can suppress melatonin production and make it difficult to fall asleep. Instead, try to disconnect from these devices at least an hour before bed and choose activities that are more relaxing and don't involve bright light.

Additionally, practicing relaxation techniques such as meditation, deep breathing, and gentle stretching can be extremely beneficial in relaxing the body and calming the mind before bed. Meditation and mindfulness can help reduce stress and anxiety, allowing you to enter a state of deep relaxation. Deep breathing can calm the nervous system, lower the heart rate and help relieve tension in the body. Gentle stretches, such as evening yoga, can release accumulated tension in muscles and promote physical relaxation.

Try different relaxation practices and identify the ones that work best for you. The important thing is to find the ones that help relax both your body and mind, preparing you for a peaceful and restorative night's sleep. By incorporating relaxing rituals into your bedtime routine, you'll be signaling your body and mind that it's time to rest, easing the transition to sleep and improving the quality of your night's rest.

## *The impact of diet and exercise on sleep quality*

### Food for healthy sleep

Food plays a key role in sleep quality. What we eat and drink throughout the day can affect our energy levels, our ability to relax and, consequently, our quality of sleep. Therefore, adopting a proper diet can contribute to healthy and restorative sleep.

One of the main recommendations for eating healthy sleep is to avoid heavy meals, especially before bedtime. Consuming a large amount of foods high in fat, sugar and complex carbohydrates before bed can overload the digestive system and make it difficult to sleep. It is preferable to eat lighter and more balanced meals at night, avoiding slow-digesting foods that can cause stomach discomfort and acid reflux.

Choosing foods that promote sleep can be beneficial. Foods rich in tryptophan, an amino acid precursor of serotonin and melatonin, are especially recommended. Serotonin is a neurotransmitter that plays an important role in regulating sleep and mood, while melatonin is the hormone responsible for regulating the sleep-wake cycle. Foods like milk, yogurt, nuts, seeds, legumes, and poultry are good sources of tryptophan and can help promote healthy sleep.

Magnesium also plays an important role in sleep, as it is involved in processes related to nervous system regulation and muscle relaxation. Foods rich in magnesium, such as dark leafy greens, almonds, avocados, bananas and fish such as salmon and tuna, can be included in the diet to help with quality sleep.

It is important to limit the consumption of substances that can interfere with sleep. Caffeine, found in coffee, tea, soda and chocolate, is a stimulant that can disrupt falling asleep and impair the quality of sleep. It is recommended to avoid caffeine consumption at least four to six hours before bedtime. Alcohol, although it may initially cause drowsiness, can interrupt sleep during the night and impair the quality of sleep. It is preferable to limit alcohol consumption and avoid consumption close to bedtime. Nicotine, present in tobacco products, is a stimulant that can disrupt sleep. Quitting smoking or avoiding tobacco use before bed can have a positive impact on sleep quality.

Keeping a food diary can be helpful in identifying which foods may be interfering with your sleep. Try making adjustments to your diet and see how your body responds.

A balanced diet geared towards healthy sleep, combined with other appropriate sleep habits, such as a regular routine, a conducive sleeping environment and relaxation practices, can significantly contribute to improving the quality of your sleep. So, when planning your meals, consider including foods that promote restful sleep and avoiding those that might get in the way. Over time, you'll discover which foods work best for you, and you'll be able to enjoy eating that supports your sleep and overall well-being.

## Physical exercise and sleep

Regular exercise plays a significant role in promoting healthy, quality sleep. The practice of physical activities brings a number of benefits to sleep, including increasing the duration and efficiency of sleep, as well as generally improving the quality of night's rest.

One of the main benefits of regular exercise is the promotion of relaxation and stress reduction. During exercise, the body releases endorphins, neurotransmitters that help relieve muscle tension and promote a sense of well-being. This can contribute to lower levels of anxiety and stress, facilitating the process of relaxation before going to bed and favoring sleep induction.

Regular exercise helps regulate the body's circadian rhythm, which is essential for quality sleep. Exposure to natural light during outdoor exercise helps to synchronize the internal biological clock, helping to regulate sleep-wake. Therefore, practicing outdoor physical activity, preferably in the morning or afternoon, can be especially beneficial for sleep.

As for the ideal time for exercise, it is recommended to avoid intense physical activity too close to bedtime. Intense exercise can raise your body temperature, increase your heart rate, and stimulate your nervous system, making it more difficult to transition to sleep. Therefore, it is preferable to schedule your exercise sessions at least a few hours before bedtime, allowing the body time to relax and calm down before preparing for the night's rest.

However, it is worth noting that each person is unique and may react differently to exercise before bed. Some people may benefit from lighter exercises, such as yoga or stretching, closer to bedtime, as these activities promote relaxation and the release of muscle tension. It's important to pay attention to your body's signals and determine what time of day and what type of exercise works best for you.

It is always recommended to consult a healthcare professional, such as a physician or physical educator, before beginning any exercise program, especially if you have any pre-existing health conditions. These professionals can advise on the appropriate type and intensity of exercise, taking into account your individual needs.

Therefore, when incorporating physical exercise into your routine, try to do it consistently and regularly. Find activities that you enjoy and that are compatible with your fitness level. Give preference to aerobic activities such as walking, running, swimming, dancing or cycling, which promote an increase in heart rate and a greater release of endorphins. Remember to time the exercise so that it fits well into your routine and allows your body enough time to relax and prepare for a restful night's sleep.

By combining a regular exercise routine with other healthy sleep habits, such as proper sleep hygiene and a conducive sleeping environment, you will be taking an important step towards improving the quality of your sleep and promoting a balanced and healthy lifestyle.

*Managing stress and anxiety before bed*

Stress management strategies

Stress management strategies play a key role in promoting healthy, restorative sleep. Chronic stress can interfere with sleep, making it difficult to fall asleep, causing frequent awakenings during the night, and impairing the overall quality of sleep. Therefore, adopting effective stress management techniques can help relax your mind and body, making it easier to transition into a peaceful sleep state.

One of the most effective approaches to stress management is the regular practice of relaxation techniques. Deep breathing is a simple yet powerful technique that can help reduce stress and anxiety. Breathing deeply and slowly, paying attention to the inhalation and exhalation, calms the nervous system, lowers the heart rate and promotes a feeling of relaxation. Meditation is also a proven practice to reduce stress. It involves focusing attention on the present moment, calming the mind, and cultivating serenity. There are several meditation techniques available, such as mindfulness meditation, which can be practiced both before bed and throughout the day to promote relaxation and mental clarity.

Practicing yoga can also be beneficial for managing stress and promoting healthy sleep.

Yoga combines gentle movement and stretching with breathing techniques and mental concentration. This combination helps to relax the body and mind, relieving the stress accumulated throughout the day. Practicing yoga before bed can be especially helpful in preparing the body for sleep, releasing muscle tension and promoting deep relaxation.

Another important strategy for managing stress is to set aside time for reflection, planning, and problem solving throughout the day. Often, worries and intrusive thoughts can arise when we are trying to sleep, damaging the quality of sleep. By setting aside a specific time during the day to address these issues, such as writing them down in a reflection notebook or making a to-do list, you can free your mind from worries before bed. This practice allows you to organize your thoughts and feel more prepared to face the challenges of the next day, providing a sense of calm and tranquility before bed.

Using gratitude journals or taking notes to release thoughts and emotions before bed can be a helpful strategy for managing stress. Writing about positive experiences, things you're grateful for, and emotions you need to express can help reduce stress and promote a more relaxed state of mind. This practice allows you to put your thoughts on paper, freeing them from the mind and facilitating the transition to a state of peaceful sleep.

By adopting these stress management strategies, you'll be giving your body and mind the tools it needs to relax, reduce anxiety, and promote quality sleep.

## Dealing with Nocturnal Anxiety

Dealing with nighttime anxiety is essential to promoting restful, restorative sleep. Anxiety can often arise or intensify during the night, making it difficult to relax and fall asleep. Fortunately, there are effective strategies to help calm the mind and reduce anxiety before bed.

One of the most effective approaches is to develop a relaxing bedtime routine. This involves establishing a set of calming, relaxing activities that signal your body and mind that it's time to relax and prepare for sleep. It could include activities like taking a warm bath, reading a book, listening to soft music, or practicing relaxation techniques like deep breathing. These activities help create a peaceful and relaxing environment, providing a smooth transition to sleep.

Anxiety reduction practices, such as mindfulness, can be extremely helpful in combating nighttime anxiety. Mindfulness involves directing attention to the present moment, cultivating mindfulness and non-judgmental awareness of the thoughts, emotions and sensations of the moment. The regular practice of mindfulness helps to calm the mind, reduce rumination and decrease emotional reactivity, contributing to a state of relaxation conducive to sleep. Incorporating mindfulness techniques before bed, such as mindfulness meditation or mindfulness of breathing, can help calm anxiety and prepare the mind for peaceful sleep.

Positive visualizations can be helpful in reducing nighttime anxiety. This technique involves creating positive and comforting mental images, such as a peaceful and serene place, a happy moment, or a relaxing situation. By viewing these images, you can feel calmer and more secure, alleviating anxiety and creating a mental environment conducive to sleep. Practicing positive visualizations regularly before bed can help train the mind to enter a state of deep relaxation and promote restful sleep.

However, if nighttime anxiety persists and significantly interferes with your sleep quality and your daily life, it is important to seek professional support. Cognitive behavioral therapy (CBT) is an effective therapeutic approach to treating anxiety and sleep disorders. A trained CBT therapist can help you identify and modify negative thinking patterns, develop healthy coping skills, and learn specific techniques for dealing with nighttime anxiety. Cognitive-behavioral therapy can provide additional support and personalized strategies for coping with anxiety, helping to restore healthy, balanced sleep.

***

Sleep hygiene plays a crucial role in promoting healthy sleep and improving overall well-being. It involves adopting a series of practices and habits that create the ideal conditions for a good night's sleep. By emphasizing the importance of sleep hygiene, you are investing in your rest and your physical, mental and emotional well-being.

One of the main recommendations for proper sleep hygiene is to create a consistent sleep routine. This involves establishing regular times to go to bed and wake up every day, including weekends. Maintaining a consistent sleep routine helps synchronize your body clock, making it easier to fall asleep and wake up. Also, having a relaxing sleep routine before bed can help prepare your body and mind for sleep. This could include activities such as taking a warm bath, reading a book, practicing relaxation techniques or meditation. By creating a relaxing bedtime routine, you signal your body that it's time to rest, helping to induce sleep more effectively.

Paying attention to your sleep environment is essential to promoting good quality sleep. A suitable sleeping environment should be cool, dark, quiet and comfortable. Make sure your bedroom is well ventilated and at a pleasant temperature, as too hot or cold can interfere with sleep. Use curtains or blinds to block outside light and minimize noise as much as possible, using ear plugs or white noise machines if necessary. Investing in a mattress and pillows that are comfortable and tailored to your individual preferences also makes for a more restful night's sleep.

It is important to consider the impact of diet, exercise, stress and anxiety management on sleep quality. A balanced and healthy diet can positively influence sleep. Avoiding heavy meals and stimulating foods before bed can help make it easier to fall asleep. On the other hand, the regular practice of physical exercises has shown significant benefits in the quality of sleep, as long as it is not performed too close to bedtime. Exercise helps reduce anxiety, relieve stress, and promote deeper, more restful sleep.

Managing stress and anxiety is also key to improving sleep quality. Stress reduction practices such as breathing techniques, meditation and yoga can calm the mind and body, preparing them for peaceful sleep. In addition, it is important to identify and address sources of stress and anxiety in your daily life, either through self-care activities such as relaxing hobbies or seeking professional support such as cognitive behavioral therapy.

By emphasizing the importance of sleep hygiene, you are acknowledging that the quality of your sleep directly affects your overall well-being. By adopting a consistent and relaxing sleep routine, caring for your sleep environment, considering food, exercise, and stress and anxiety management, you are investing in your sleep and well-being.

Each person is unique and may require individual adjustments to their sleep routine. So explore and experiment with different strategies to find what works best for you. With dedication and persistence, you can improve the quality of your sleep and enjoy a healthier, more balanced life.

# Improving the Sleep Environment

*Creating an environment conducive to sleep: mattress, pillows, temperature, light and noise*

## Choosing the right mattress

Choosing the right mattress is of paramount importance to ensuring a comfortable and quality sleep. An inadequate mattress can negatively affect your comfort, support and, consequently, the quality of your sleep. Therefore, when considering the choice of a mattress, it is important to consider several individual factors.

One of the main aspects to be considered is the firmness level of the mattress. The ideal firmness varies from person to person, as everyone has their own personal preferences. Some prefer a firmer mattress, while others prefer a softer mattress. It's important to find a balance that provides adequate support for your spine, keeping it aligned while providing comfort and pressure relief at your body's touch points.

In addition to firmness, it's crucial to consider your body's specific needs. If you have back pain, for example, a mattress that offers adequate support for your spine can be critical. In this case, a medium to firm mattress may be more appropriate. However, it is important to note that each person is unique, and it is essential to seek medical advice if you have specific concerns related to back problems or back pain.

Another factor to consider is the presence of allergies. For allergic people, it is important to choose a hypoallergenic mattress, which is resistant to dust mites, bacteria and other allergens. In addition, mattresses made with natural materials, such as organic latex or organic cotton, can be an interesting option for those looking to avoid chemicals or synthetic materials that can trigger allergic reactions.

When choosing a mattress, it's also critical to consider the proper size for your individual needs. Make sure the mattress is spacious enough for you to move around comfortably during the night, especially if you share a bed with a partner. Choosing the right mattress size can prevent discomfort and sleep interruptions due to insufficient space.

Finally, it's important to mention that choosing the right mattress may require a trial period. Many stores offer the option of testing the mattress for a few weeks or months, allowing you to gauge comfort and support before making a final decision. Take this opportunity to try out different mattress types and see how well they fit your body and your individual needs.

In summary, choosing the right mattress is a personal and individualized decision. Consider your firmness preference, specific needs such as back pain or allergies, and the proper size to ensure quality, comfortable sleep.

## Selecting the Perfect Pillows

Choosing the right pillows plays a key role in maintaining proper neck and head posture while sleeping. An inadequate pillow can result in discomfort, stiffness and even neck and shoulder pain. Therefore, when selecting a pillow, it is important to consider several aspects, taking into account your personal preferences and individual needs.

There are several types of pillows available on the market, each with unique characteristics.

Feather pillows, for example, are soft and conformable, providing gentle support for the head and neck. On the other hand, memory foam pillows, also known as memory foam pillows, adapt to the shape of the body, offering personalized support and pressure relief. Latex pillows are known for their durability and strength, as well as offering firm and stable support.

When choosing a pillow, consider your personal preferences for height and firmness. The height of the pillow must be adequate to keep the head and neck aligned with the spine, avoiding tension and pain. If you sleep on your side, a taller pillow may be needed to fill the gap between your shoulder and head. If you sleep on your back or on your back, a medium to low height pillow may be more suitable for maintaining a neutral neck position.

Pillow firmness is also an important consideration. Some prefer a firm pillow for added support, while others prefer a softer pillow for added comfort. Keep in mind that ideal firmness may vary based on your personal preferences and individual needs. It's important to test different options and consider your comfort when choosing pillow firmness.

Take into account the materials of the pillow. Some materials are more breathable and provide better ventilation, contributing to a cooler sleeping environment. For example, feather pillows can allow for better air circulation, while memory foam pillows can retain more heat. Consider your preferences for breathability and sleeping temperature when choosing pillow material.

It's important to remember that choosing the ideal pillow can vary from person to person. What works for one person may not be suitable for another. Therefore, it is recommended to experiment with different types of pillows and observe how your body responds to them. Some stores offer the option of testing pillows for a period of time before making a final decision.

In short, selecting the ideal pillow is a personal and individualized decision. Consider proper neck and head posture while sleeping, the different types of pillows available, and your personal preferences for height, firmness, and materials. By choosing a pillow that provides adequate support and comfort while sleeping, you will be contributing to a better quality of sleep and to your overall well-being.

## Regulating the room temperature

Room temperature plays a significant role in sleep quality. An environment with the right temperature can promote relaxation and help the body enter a state of deep, restorative sleep. Therefore, it is important to create an environment with a comfortable temperature to optimize sleep.

The ideal temperature range for comfortable sleep varies from person to person, but is generally between 18°C and 22°C. This range provides a balance between warming and cooling the body during sleep. However, it is important to note that each individual has their own personal preferences and that thermal comfort may vary according to individual factors, such as metabolism and sensitivity to heat or cold.

To adjust the room temperature, there are several strategies that can be adopted. During the warmer months, using fans or air conditioning can help reduce the temperature and keep the room cool. Make sure the fan or air conditioner is properly positioned, facing away from the bed, to avoid direct drafts on the body.

In the colder months, heaters or central heating systems can be used to keep the room warm. It is important to ensure that the temperature does not get too high, as this can cause discomfort and interfere with sleep quality. A slightly cool but cozy environment is generally preferable.

In addition, it is recommended to use suitable bedding for each season. During the summer, opt for cotton sheets or light, breathable fabrics, which help regulate body temperature and promote a feeling of freshness. In winter, choose warmer materials, such as flannel or thermal fabrics, to ensure comfort and warmth.

Another tip is to pay attention to your own signs of thermal comfort. If you frequently wake up feeling too hot or too cold, you may need to adjust your room temperature or make changes to your bedding.

Temperature control is not just limited to the environment. Body temperature also plays an important role in sleep. Take a warm bath before bed to help you relax and allow your body temperature to gradually decrease, preparing your body for sleep.

In short, creating an environment with the right temperature is essential to promote peaceful and restorative sleep. Experiment with different temperature ranges to find the one that best suits your individual needs and preferences. Use strategies such as using fans, air conditioning or heaters to adjust the room temperature. In addition, choose appropriate bedding for each season and pay attention to your own signs of thermal comfort.

## Dealing with light and noise

A dark, quiet bedroom is essential for promoting quality sleep. Excessive light and noise can interfere with your ability to fall asleep, stay asleep, and achieve deep rest. Therefore, adopting strategies to block light and reduce noise is essential to create an environment conducive to sleep.

Exposure to light before bed can interfere with the production of the sleep hormone melatonin, which helps regulate circadian rhythms and induce sleep. Blocking out excessive light in the environment can help signal the body that it's time to rest. One option is to use blackout curtains, which effectively block outside light from entering. These curtains are made of a special fabric that prevents the passage of light, keeping the room dark and providing a more peaceful sleep. Also, using sleep masks or eye shields can help block out unwanted light, especially if you are having trouble completely darkening your room.

Noise can also interfere with sleep quality, making it more superficial and fragmented. To reduce noise disturbance, the use of noise suppressors such as ear plugs or white noise machines is recommended. Earplugs are small foam or silicone devices that fit in the ear canal, decreasing the perception of external sounds. They are especially useful for blocking out ambient noise, such as traffic, neighbors, or roommates snoring. White noise machines emit soft, steady sounds that help mask unwanted noise and create a more peaceful sleep environment.

In addition to light and noise blocking strategies, it is important to evaluate other factors that may be interfering with sleep quality. For example, check the bedroom for unwanted light sources, such as lights from electronic devices or digital clocks, and turn them off or cover them up at night. Also, consider reducing indoor noise, such as using headphones to listen to relaxing music or adopting relaxation practices to calm the mind before bed.

## *The importance of darkness and tips for blocking out excessive light*

### The role of darkness in sleep regulation

Darkness plays a crucial role in regulating sleep, mainly through its influence on the production of the sleep hormone melatonin. Melatonin is secreted by the pineal gland at night and helps regulate our body's circadian cycle, or biological rhythm. It plays a key role in promoting deep, restorative sleep.

Exposure to light, especially artificial light, at night can interfere with melatonin production, disrupting circadian rhythms and negatively affecting sleep. Artificial light, such as that emitted by electronic devices (such as smartphones, tablets and televisions) and indoor lights, contains a higher proportion of blue light, which is particularly effective at suppressing melatonin production. This is because blue light is perceived by our visual system as a sign that it is daytime and therefore inhibits melatonin production, disrupting the natural induction of sleep.

Melatonin suppression due to exposure to light at night can lead to difficulty falling asleep, fragmented and less restful sleep. Furthermore, this circadian rhythm disruption may have broader health impacts, affecting mood, cognition, the immune system, and hormone regulation.

Therefore, it is important to create an environment conducive to sleep, where darkness is prioritized. This can be done through the use of blackout curtains, blinds or shutters that effectively block outside light. In addition, it is recommended to avoid using electronic devices before bed, at least one hour before bedtime, to reduce exposure to blue light. If it is necessary to use these devices, it is advisable to use applications or settings that filter blue light, helping to minimize its impact on sleep.

By creating a dark environment before bed, you are sending a signal to your body that it is time to rest, allowing melatonin production to take place properly. This contributes to deeper, more restorative, quality sleep.

Importantly, darkness is not only important during nighttime sleep, but also during daytime naps. For efficient sleep, it is recommended to look for dark and silent environments, even during daytime naps, to make the most of the benefits of rest.

## Strategies to block out excessive light

There are several effective strategies for blocking out excessive light and creating a dark environment that promotes quality sleep. These strategies are especially important for those who have difficulty falling asleep or maintaining a deep sleep due to the presence of unwanted light. Here are some suggestions for blocking out excessive light:

**Use of blackout curtains or blinds:** Investing in blackout curtains or blinds is an excellent way to effectively block out outside light. These curtains are made of opaque materials that prevent the passage of light, making the room significantly darker. By closing them completely, you can create an ideal environment for sleep, even during the day.

**Removing or turning off electronic devices with bright lights:** Many electronic devices, such as smartphones, tablets, digital watches and televisions, have bright lights that can interfere with the quality of sleep. It is important to remove these devices from the bedroom or turn them off before going to sleep to avoid exposure to artificial light. If it is necessary to keep any devices in the room, you can cover the lights with opaque stickers or dark masking tape to reduce their glare.

**Use of sleep masks or blindfolds:** Sleep masks, also known as blindfolds, are a convenient and effective option for blocking outside light. They are made of soft and comfortable materials that fit over the eyes, completely covering them. By using a sleep mask, you create a physical barrier between your eyes and ambient light, promoting a dark and sleep-friendly environment.

In addition to these strategies, it is important to evaluate other light sources in the bedroom and take steps to minimize them. For example, you can turn off or cover lights on electronic devices such as routers, chargers, or digital alarm clocks. It is also recommended to invest in light switches with dimming control, so that you can adjust the ambient lighting according to your needs.

*The role of technology in sleep quality: electronic devices, blue light and strategies to minimize its negative impact*

## Understanding the influence of technology on sleep

Understanding the influence of technology on sleep is critical to improving sleep quality and promoting adequate rest. Exposure to blue light emitted by electronic devices, such as smartphones, tablets and computers, has been shown to be one of the main factors that interfere with sleep.

Blue light, present in large amounts in these screens, is especially effective in suppressing the production of melatonin, the sleep hormone. Exposure to blue light at night confuses the body's biological clock, erroneously indicating that it's still daytime and inhibiting melatonin production, which can make it difficult to fall asleep and affect the quality of sleep.

Emotionally charged or stimulating content present in many apps, games or movies can also have a negative impact on sleep. These types of content can activate the nervous system, increase arousal, and make it difficult to transition into a state of proper relaxation before bed. The result is an agitated mind, difficulty shutting off thoughts, and less restful sleep.

To minimize the negative effects of technology on sleep, some measures can be adopted. The first is to limit the use of electronic devices before bedtime, especially about an hour before bedtime. This allows the brain to enter a state of relaxation and prepare for sleep. It is recommended to establish a nightly ritual that does not involve the use of these devices, such as reading a book, taking a relaxing bath or practicing relaxation techniques.

There are apps and settings available that can help reduce your exposure to the blue light emitted by electronic devices. These tools filter blue light and change the screen's color temperature to warmer tones, reducing the negative impact on the circadian rhythm.

Another option is to wear blue light blocking glasses, which filter out harmful light emitted by electronic devices, helping to protect natural melatonin production and promote more restful sleep.

## Strategies to minimize the negative impact of technology on sleep

To minimize the negative impact of technology on sleep, it is essential to adopt strategies that help reduce exposure to blue light emitted by electronic devices. Here are some effective approaches to minimizing technology's impact on sleep:

Implementing a "disconnect time": Set aside at least an hour before bed to disconnect from electronic devices. Avoid the use of smartphones, tablets, computers and televisions during this time. Instead, choose relaxing, technology-free activities like reading a book, listening to quiet music, practicing relaxation techniques, writing in a journal, or talking with family. This "disconnect time" helps prepare the brain and body for sleep by reducing stimulation and allowing the mind to relax.

Enabling night mode and using blue light filters: Many electronic devices have a night mode that changes the color temperature of the screen, reducing blue light emission. Activating this function helps reduce exposure to blue light before bedtime. Additionally, there are apps and filters available that can be installed on electronic devices to reduce blue light emission. These tools adjust the hue of the screen, making it warmer and less stimulating to the eyes.

Establishing a technology-free area in the bedroom: Reserving the bedroom only for activities related to sleep and relaxation is an effective strategy. Keep the sleeping area clear of electronic devices such as smartphones, tablets and televisions. Also, avoid keeping these devices next to your bed at night. By creating a technology-free area in the bedroom, you help to associate the environment with rest and relaxation, contributing to a better quality of sleep.

***

Creating a suitable sleep environment plays a key role in promoting good quality sleep.

Small changes to your environment can make a big difference in your sleep and overall well-being. Here are some essential aspects to consider for an ideal sleep environment:

**Choosing suitable mattresses and pillows:** A proper mattress and pillow are essential to provide comfort and support while sleeping. The right choice depends on individual preferences and specific needs, such as spinal alignment, support for problem areas or allergies. It is important to invest in quality products that meet your needs and provide a comfortable sleeping environment.

**Temperature regulation:** Room temperature can significantly influence sleep quality. Most people tend to sleep better in a cool room with a temperature between 18°C and 22°C. Try adjusting the room temperature according to your personal preferences. This may involve using fans, air conditioning, heaters or opening windows to allow adequate air circulation.

**Excessive light blocking:** Darkness is a crucial element for quality sleep. Exposure to bright light, especially the blue light emitted by electronic devices, can suppress the production of melatonin, the sleep hormone. Use blackout curtains or blinds that effectively block light from entering the room. If necessary, use sleep masks or eye shields to create a dark, sleep-friendly environment.

**Reduced exposure to technology before bed:** Exposure to blue light emitted by electronic devices such as smartphones, tablets and computers can interfere with sleep quality. Blue light suppresses melatonin production, making it difficult to induce sleep. To improve sleep quality, avoid using these devices at least one hour before bed. Instead, opt for relaxing activities such as reading, meditation, a warm bath, or relaxation techniques.

By creating an adequate sleep environment, you are establishing the ideal conditions for good quality sleep. Small changes like choosing the right mattress and pillows, regulating the temperature, blocking excessive light, and reducing exposure to technology can make a big difference in the quality of your sleep and your overall well-being. By adopting these practices, you will be investing in your sleep and reaping the benefits of restorative rest.

# Relaxation and Meditation Techniques

*Relaxation practices to prepare the body and mind for sleep*

Hot shower

Taking a hot bath before bed can be an effective strategy to relax your muscles and reduce tension built up throughout the day. The heat from the hot water helps to dilate blood vessels, improving circulation and promoting a feeling of relaxation throughout the body.

In addition to the physical benefit, adding relaxing essential oils, such as lavender, to bath water can enhance the calming effect. Lavender is known for its relaxing and aromatic properties, which can help calm the mind and prepare the body for sleep. The soothing, comforting scent of lavender has been linked to reducing anxiety, stress and agitation, creating an environment conducive to peaceful sleep.

By taking a warm bath with relaxing essential oils, you can enjoy the therapeutic benefits of both the warm water and the soothing scents. This combination helps relax your muscles, relieve stress and tension, and prepare your body and mind for a restful, restful night's sleep.

Be sure to properly dilute essential oils in a carrier oil before adding them to the bathwater, following the proper instructions.

Adding a warm bath to your nightly routine can be an enjoyable way to relax and prepare for a good night's sleep. Enjoy the physical and mental benefits of this practice, allowing yourself to slow down and enjoy a moment of self-care before giving yourself over to rest.

## Massage

Massage is an effective technique for relieving muscle tension and promoting relaxation of body and mind. There are different approaches to massage, including self-massage, which you can do yourself, and massage performed by a trained professional.

Self-massage involves applying pressure and gentle strokes to areas of tension in the body. You can use your hands, fingers, or even massage accessories like rollers or balls to target specific areas. This practice can help release muscle tension built up throughout the day, promoting a sense of relaxation and well-being.

By incorporating relaxing essential oils during the massage, you can enhance the calming and therapeutic effects of the practice. Some essential oils known for their relaxing properties include lavender, chamomile, bergamot and ylang-ylang. These essential oils can be diluted with a carrier oil, such as almond or coconut oil, before being applied to the skin during a massage. The pleasant, soothing aroma of these oils can help calm the mind and induce a feeling of deep relaxation.

However, it is important to remember that massage may not be right for everyone in all situations. Some people may have specific medical conditions that require the advice of a healthcare professional before starting any form of massage. In addition, massage performed by a trained professional can offer additional benefits, such as specific muscle manipulation techniques and relief of tension points.

Massage, whether in the form of self-massage or with the help of a professional, can be an excellent way to relax muscles, release tension and prepare the body for peaceful sleep. Experiment with different techniques and essential oils to find what works best for you, and enjoy the physical and mental benefits of this relaxation practice.

## Stretching and Gentle Yoga

Stretching and gentle yoga are great ways to relax your body and mind before bed. Gentle stretching involves slow, controlled movements stretching the muscles and releasing tension built up throughout the day. These exercises help improve flexibility, relieve muscle stress, and promote a feeling of deep relaxation.

In addition to stretching, gentle yoga is a practice that combines gentle movement, mindful breathing, and relaxation. Certain yoga poses are particularly beneficial for preparing the body for sleep. Corpse Pose (Savasana), for example, is a relaxation pose where you lie on your back, allowing your body to completely relax on the floor. This pose helps to calm the mind and release muscle tension, preparing the body for a peaceful night's sleep.

Another yoga pose that can be performed before bed is the Happy Baby Pose (Balasana). In this position, you kneel down, sit back on your heels and bend your body forward, extending your arms in front of you or at your sides. This pose gently stretches the spine, relaxes the back and shoulder muscles, and provides a feeling of comfort and relaxation.

In addition to the physical benefits, stretching and gentle yoga also help calm the mind and relax the nervous system. The emphasis on mindful breathing during these practices promotes a sense of calm and tranquility, preparing the body and mind for a restful night's sleep.

When practicing stretching and gentle yoga before bed, it's important to listen to your body and respect its limits. Don't force the movements and be present in the moment, paying attention to your breath and the sensations in your body.

Incorporating gentle stretching and yoga sessions before bed can be an effective way to relax your body, ease muscle tension, and prepare for a restful, restful night's sleep. Try different exercises and poses, find what works best for you, and enjoy the benefits of stretching and gentle yoga for your sleep and overall well-being.

*Meditation and mindfulness as tools to reduce anxiety and promote peaceful sleep*

## guided meditation

Guided meditation is a practice that involves focusing the mind on a specific object of attention, such as the breath, words or images, to calm the mind and relax the body. It is a widely used technique to reduce stress, promote relaxation and improve sleep quality.

Meditation itself has a number of mental and emotional health benefits. It helps calm a busy mind, reduce anxiety and promote an overall sense of well-being. By bringing attention to the present moment and cultivating mindfulness, meditation helps stop the constant flow of thoughts and worries, allowing the mind to rest and rejuvenate itself.

Guided meditation is especially helpful for those who are new to the practice or have difficulty meditating on their own. By following a recording, instructions or a meditation app, you are guided step by step into a state of relaxation and mindfulness. The guide's voice offers guidance and suggestions to help you relax your body, calm your mind and connect with the present moment.

Guided meditation can be done anywhere, including the comfort of your own bedroom before bed. You can find specific guided meditations for sleep and relaxation designed to help you prepare for a peaceful night's sleep. These meditations usually involve deep breathing exercises, progressive body relaxation, and calming visualizations.

Additionally, guided meditation can be a valuable tool for those who have difficulty calming their mind before bed. By focusing on the guide's voice and following the instructions, you can shift your attention from disquieting thoughts and engage with the present experience. This helps to reduce mental rumination, anxiety and agitation, creating a calm state conducive to sleep.

There are many options available for accessing guided meditations. Popular meditation apps offer a variety of guided sessions, from short five-minute meditations to longer sessions. Additionally, there are plenty of recordings available online and on streaming platforms, covering specific topics such as relaxation, sleep and stress management.

When incorporating guided meditation into your sleep routine, it's important to find a calm and peaceful environment where you can sit or lie down comfortably. Make time for practice regularly and experiment with different approaches until you find the meditations and instructions that resonate with you.

## mindfulness practice

The practice of mindfulness, or full attention, is a way of training the mind to be consciously present in the current moment, without judgment or attachment to thoughts and emotions. This practice has been shown to be effective in reducing stress and anxiety and cultivating a sense of calm and well-being.

When applied before bed, mindfulness can be especially helpful in calming the mind and preparing the body for sleep. Through mindfulness, it is possible to divert attention from the intrusive thoughts and worries that may arise at bedtime. This creates a more peaceful mental space conducive to sleep.

A common mindfulness exercise that can be practiced before bed is the body scan. In this practice, you intentionally direct your attention to different parts of your body, noticing the physical sensations present. Starting at the head and working your way down to the feet, you can pay attention to feelings of tension, heat, tingling, or any other sensation that arises. The goal is not to alter or judge these sensations, but rather to be consciously present with them, allowing the body to relax and release any built-up tension.

When practicing mindfulness, it is important to remember that the mind can wander and become distracted by thoughts. This is normal and part of the practice. When you notice that the mind has wandered away, gently bring your attention back to your body and present sensations. This training of the mind to return to the present moment helps to reduce mental rumination and anxiety before bed.

In addition to body scanning, there are many other mindfulness practices you can do before bed, such as mindful breathing, watching your thoughts without getting attached to them, and viewing relaxing images. You can find mindfulness and meditation apps that offer specific sessions for relaxation and sleep.

Practicing mindfulness before bed can be a powerful complement to promoting healthy sleep. By cultivating mindfulness and awareness in the present moment, you can reduce the stressful thoughts and worries that can disrupt sleep.

*Breathing exercises and other techniques to calm the mind before bed*

## Deep breath

Deep breathing is a simple and effective technique that can be used as a powerful tool to relax the body, calm the nervous system, and ward off anxious thoughts before bed. It involves bringing your attention to your breath and practicing slow, deep, conscious breathing.

A commonly used deep breathing exercise is belly breathing, also known as diaphragmatic breathing. To practice it, find a comfortable position, sitting or lying down. Place one hand on your chest and the other on your abdomen. Inhale slowly through your nose, filling your abdomen with air, allowing it to expand as your hand rises. Then gently exhale through your mouth, releasing all the air and allowing your abdomen to contract. Repeat this cycle of deep breathing for a few minutes, focusing on the sensation of air moving in and out of your body.

When practicing deep breathing, it's important to remember to breathe in a slow, smooth, and controlled manner, avoiding quick, shallow breaths. Deep breathing helps activate the parasympathetic nervous system, which is responsible for relaxation and stress reduction.

In addition to abdominal breathing, there are other breathing techniques that can also be helpful for relaxing before bed. One is the 4-7-8 breath, where you inhale through your nose for a count of 4, hold your breath for a count of 7, and then exhale through your mouth for a count of 8. Repeat this cycle a few times, allowing your body and mind to calm down.

By focusing on your breath during these exercises, you shift your attention away from anxious thoughts and into the present moment. Mindful breathing helps calm the mind and relax the body, preparing you for a restful night's sleep.

Additionally, practicing deep breathing exercises regularly throughout the day can help reduce general anxiety and promote a state of relaxation. Take a few minutes each day to practice these breathing techniques and reap the benefits in your sleep quality and overall well-being.

Try different deep breathing techniques and find the ones that work best for you. Practice them regularly before bed and whenever you feel the need to relax and calm your mind. Deep breathing is a simple yet powerful tool that is always there to help you find a state of tranquility and prepare for restorative sleep.

## progressive muscle relaxation

Progressive muscle relaxation is an effective technique for relieving accumulated tension and stress in the body. It involves the sequential contraction and relaxation of different muscle groups, leading to a feeling of deep relaxation and physical relaxation.

To practice progressive muscle relaxation, find a quiet, comfortable environment where you can lie down or sit in a relaxed position. Close your eyes and focus on your breathing, allowing the air to flow in and out smoothly.

Start by directing your attention to the muscles in your feet. Intentionally contract them by squeezing them for a few seconds and then release them completely by relaxing them. Note the difference between the feeling of tension and relaxation in the muscles of the feet.

Then move your attention to the leg muscles. Contract them by squeezing the thigh and calf muscles for a few seconds, then release them, allowing the tension to release. Feel the feeling of relaxation spreading through your legs.

Continue working your way through the body, directing your attention to the muscles in your abdomen, back, shoulders, arms, hands, neck, and face. In each muscle group, intentionally contract the muscles and then completely release them, releasing any built-up tension.

As you progress through your body, notice the feelings of relaxation and allow them to deepen with each release of tension. Focus on the difference between muscle tension and relaxation, allowing your entire body to surrender to a state of deep relaxation.

To assist in the practice of progressive muscle relaxation, you can use apps or recordings that guide the process step by step. These tools can provide verbal instructions for each muscle group, helping you to focus and relax even more.

Progressive muscle relaxation can be a useful technique for reducing physical and mental tension before bed. By releasing muscle tension, you create an environment more conducive to relaxation and peaceful sleep.

Practice progressive muscle relaxation regularly, either before bed or at times of stress throughout the day. With practice, you will learn to recognize and release muscle tension more effectively, promoting deeper sleep and an overall sense of well-being.

## guided views

Guided visualizations are an effective technique for inducing a state of deep relaxation and calming the mind before bed. This practice involves creating calming, positive mental images that help reduce anxiety and promote peaceful sleep.

To start a guided visualization, find a quiet spot where you can sit or lie down comfortably. Close your eyes and begin to relax your body and mind, breathing deeply and releasing any tension that is present.

Then start creating a relaxing mental image. It could be a serene spot in nature, like a sunny beach, a lush garden, or a peaceful forest. Visualize yourself in this environment, observing the details around you: the colors, sounds, smells and sensations.

Focus on all the positive aspects of this place. Feel the warm sun on your skin, the gentle breeze caressing your face, the fresh scent of nature all around you. Allow yourself to be completely involved with this image, as if you were really there.

As you explore this visualization, allow your mind to relax and drift away from stressful thoughts or worries. Focus only on the calming, positive sensations of the environment you are imagining.

To further enhance the practice of guided visualization, you can use audio recordings with detailed instructions or create your own custom visualizations. These recordings can include directions for relaxing each part of the body, describing the imagined scene, and incorporating deep breathing techniques.

By using guided visualizations before bed, you create a state of deep relaxation, which can help to calm your agitated mind and prepare your body for sleep. Guided visualization is an effective tool for taking your focus away from stressful and anxious thoughts, allowing you to enter a state of tranquility and serenity.

Practice guided imagery regularly, taking a moment before bed to engage with this technique. Over time, you will develop skills to create relaxing mental images on your own, which will allow you to use this technique whenever you feel the need to relax and calm your mind.

\*\*\*

Relaxation techniques, meditation and breathing exercises play a crucial role in preparing the body and mind for a peaceful night's sleep. These practices help reduce mental activity, calm the nervous system and relieve accumulated tension, allowing you to disconnect from the worries of the day and enter a state of deep relaxation.

By experimenting with different relaxation techniques, meditation, and breathing exercises, you may find the ones that work best for you. Each person is unique and may respond differently to different practices. Some people may benefit from mindfulness meditation, while others find that deep breathing is more effective for them. It's important to explore and discover which techniques resonate with you the best.

By regularly incorporating these techniques into your sleep routine, you create a habit that gradually prepares your body and mind for a smooth transition to sleep. The regular practice of these techniques helps to decrease mental activity, reduce anxiety and calm the nervous system, providing an ideal state of relaxation for sleep.

In addition to promoting peaceful sleep, relaxation techniques, meditation and breathing exercises also have significant benefits for overall quality of life. They help reduce stress, improve concentration, increase mental clarity and strengthen the ability to deal with emotions. These practices can help cultivate a sense of calm and balance in your daily life.

It is important to keep in mind that each person may have different preferences regarding relaxation and meditation techniques. What works for one person may not work the same way for another. Therefore, it is encouraged to experiment with different approaches, techniques and practices to find the ones that are most effective and enjoyable for you.

By incorporating these practices into your nightly routine, you'll be laying a solid foundation for quality sleep and a better quality of life in general. Remember to take time out for yourself to relax and take care of your mental health. With patience and persistence, you can develop a practice that fits your individual needs, helping you to achieve restful sleep and a more balanced, healthy life.

# Supplements and Natural Remedies

*Natural alternatives to aid sleep, such as calming teas and essential oils*

## calming teas

Calming teas are a natural and popular option to help relax the body and mind before bed. There are several herbs known for their relaxing properties that can be brewed as teas and consumed as part of an evening routine to promote peaceful sleep and relieve stress and anxiety.

One of the best known herbs for this purpose is chamomile. Chamomile has been widely used as a natural remedy to calm nerves and induce sleep. It contains natural compounds that have calming effects on the body, reducing anxiety and promoting feelings of relaxation.

Another commonly used herb is lemon balm, also known as melissa. Lemon balm has mild sedative properties that help calm the mind and relax the muscles. In addition to its relaxing effects, lemon balm can also help relieve symptoms of stress, anxiety and sleep disorders.

Valerian is a plant popularly known for its calming properties. It has been used for centuries as a natural remedy to promote sleep and relieve anxiety. Valerian has compounds that help relax the nervous system, reducing tension and making it easier to fall asleep.

Lavender is an herb known for its soothing, relaxing scent. It has sedative properties that help reduce stress and anxiety, promoting a state of relaxation conducive to sleep. Lavender can also help alleviate symptoms of insomnia and improve sleep quality.

For best results when preparing and consuming calming teas, it is recommended to follow some guidelines. It is important to use hot, but not boiling, water to preserve the medicinal properties of the herbs. Generally, one tablespoon of dried herbs to one cup of water is adequate. Let the herbs steep for about 5 to 10 minutes to allow the active compounds to be released into the water. If you wish, you can sweeten the tea with honey or a natural sweetener.

It is important to note that each person may respond differently to calming teas. Some people may feel the calming effects right away, while others may need some time to get used to it and experience the benefits. In addition, it is recommended to avoid excessive consumption of soothing teas, especially if you are pregnant, breastfeeding or taking medication, to avoid possible interactions.

Soothing teas can be a relaxing and healthy addition to your nighttime routine. By combining these herbs with other relaxation techniques, such as meditation, deep breathing, or reading a book, you can create an environment conducive to sleep and promote peaceful rest. Try different types of calming teas and discover which ones work best for you, enjoying the benefits of these natural herbs to relax, relieve stress and promote restful sleep.

## Essential oils

Essential oils are concentrated plant extracts that have therapeutic and aromatic properties. Some essential oils are known for their relaxing properties and can be used to promote peaceful and restful sleep. Some examples of essential oils with these properties include lavender, chamomile, and sandalwood.

Lavender is one of the most popular and widely used essential oils to promote calm and relaxation. Its soft, floral aroma has relaxing effects on the nervous system, helping to reduce stress and anxiety. Lavender is also known for its sedative properties, which can make it easier to fall asleep and improve sleep quality.

Chamomile is another essential oil with relaxing and calming properties. Its sweet, herbal aroma has soothing effects on the nervous system, helping to calm the mind and ease tension. Chamomile can also be helpful in reducing anxiety and promoting peaceful sleep.

Sandalwood is an essential oil known for its relaxing and aromatic properties. Its earthy and woody aroma helps create a peaceful atmosphere conducive to relaxation. Sandalwood can also help reduce stress and promote deep, restful sleep.

There are several ways to use essential oils to promote sleep. Aromatherapy is one of the most popular ways, which involves using a diffuser to disperse aromatic molecules into the air. Inhaling the aroma of essential oils can have calming and relaxing effects, preparing your body and mind for sleep. In addition, essential oils can be diluted in a carrier oil and applied through gentle massages, providing a relaxing effect for both body and mind. Another option is to add a few drops of essential oils to the bath water, allowing the aroma to be absorbed into the skin and inhaled during the shower.

When using essential oils, it is important to consider some precautions. First, make sure you are purchasing high quality essential oils from reputable sources. Also, always follow recommended dosage instructions and avoid overuse. Some essential oils can be irritating to the skin or cause allergic reactions, so it is recommended that you do a sensitivity test before using a new essential oil. It is important to respect individual preferences and needs, and if any adverse reactions occur, discontinue use.

Essential oils can be a relaxing and aromatic addition to your nighttime routine. By experimenting with different essential oils and methods of use, you can discover which scents and techniques work best for you, promoting restful, restful sleep. Remember to choose quality essential oils, use the proper dosages, and consider your own needs and preferences for best results.

## *Dietary supplements that can promote healthy sleep*

### Melatonin

Melatonin is a hormone naturally produced by the human body, secreted by the pineal gland, located in the brain. Its main function is to regulate the sleep-wake cycle, helping to induce sleep and synchronize the circadian rhythm, which is the body's internal clock responsible for determining sleep and wake patterns throughout the day.

Melatonin production is influenced by exposure to light. Normally, melatonin production increases as the light dims, preparing the body for sleep. During the night, melatonin peaks, promoting deep, restorative sleep. At dawn, with exposure to sunlight, melatonin production decreases, helping to maintain wakefulness.

Melatonin supplementation has been widely used as an option to help induce sleep, especially in cases of insomnia or circadian rhythm dysregulation. Melatonin supplements are available in pill, capsule, or liquid form, and are often recommended for short-term use.

When using melatonin supplements, it is important to consider some important information. First, it is recommended to consult a healthcare professional before starting supplementation to determine the proper dosage and duration of use. Dosages may vary depending on age, individual needs and health conditions.

In addition, it is important to follow the guidelines regarding the time of consumption. Melatonin is usually taken about 30 minutes to an hour before bed to allow the body to absorb and utilize the hormone properly. This may vary depending on the specific supplement instructions and physician recommendations.

It is also essential to be aware of possible interactions with other medications. Melatonin can interact with certain medications, such as blood thinners, blood pressure medications, and medications that affect the immune system. It's critical to tell your doctor about all medications you're taking, including supplements, to avoid unwanted interactions.

Although melatonin is considered safe for most people, some precautions should be taken. Pregnant or nursing women, children, and people with certain health conditions should consult a healthcare professional before using melatonin.

It is important to remember that melatonin is not a substitute for good sleep hygiene and healthy sleep habits. It can be a useful tool to help adjust the circadian rhythm and promote sleep induction, but it is critical to take a holistic approach to improving sleep quality, including creating a consistent sleep routine, a suitable sleeping environment, the practice of relaxation techniques and the adoption of healthy lifestyle habits.

In summary, melatonin is a hormone naturally produced by the body to regulate sleep and circadian rhythm. Melatonin supplementation may be an option to help induce sleep and adjust the circadian rhythm, but it is important to consult a health professional, follow the appropriate dosages, consider the times of consumption and be aware of possible interactions with other medications. It is essential to take a comprehensive approach to promoting healthy sleep, including sleep hygiene habits, relaxation techniques and a balanced lifestyle.

## tryptophan and magnesium

Tryptophan and Magnesium are nutrients that play important roles in promoting healthy sleep and relaxing the body and mind.

Tryptophan is an essential amino acid, which means that it is not produced by the body and must be obtained through food. Tryptophan is a precursor to serotonin, a neurotransmitter that plays a crucial role in regulating mood, sleep and general well-being. Serotonin is converted into melatonin, the hormone responsible for regulating the sleep-wake cycle.

Tryptophan-rich foods include:

- Lean meats such as chicken breast and turkey
- Fish, such as salmon and tuna
- Eggs
- Dairy products, such as milk and yogurt
- Legumes, such as beans, lentils and chickpeas
- Nuts and seeds, such as almonds, cashews and pumpkin seeds

In addition to obtaining tryptophan through their diet, some people may consider supplemental tryptophan, especially if they have specific deficiencies or conditions that may interfere with proper absorption of this amino acid. However, it is important to consult a healthcare professional before starting supplementation, as dosage and duration of use may vary according to individual needs.

Another important nutrient for sleep is magnesium. Magnesium plays an essential role in regulating the nervous system and reducing stress and anxiety, promoting muscle and mental relaxation. In addition, magnesium is involved in the production of melatonin.

Dietary sources rich in magnesium include:

- Green leafy vegetables like spinach and kale
- Nuts and seeds, such as almonds, cashews, pumpkin seeds, and sunflower seeds
- Whole grains such as oats and quinoa
- Legumes, such as black beans, pinto beans, and lentils
- Bananas

As with tryptophan, some people may consider magnesium supplementation, especially if they have specific deficiencies or difficulties obtaining adequate amounts through their diet. However, it is important to consult a healthcare professional to determine the proper dosage and to consider possible interactions with other medications.

It is worth noting that while tryptophan and magnesium supplementation may be beneficial for some people, obtaining these nutrients through a balanced and varied diet is always the best approach. In addition, it is important to remember that the overall quality of the diet and healthy lifestyle play a key role in promoting sleep and well-being. Therefore, it is recommended to take a holistic approach, including a balanced diet, regular exercise, relaxation techniques and a consistent sleep routine, to obtain the best results.

## *Considerations about the use of sleeping pills and their possible consequences*

## sleeping pills

Sleeping drugs such as benzodiazepines and zolpidem are prescribed to treat sleep disorders, especially in cases of severe insomnia or specific disorders that significantly affect quality of life. These drugs belong to the class of sedatives and hypnotics and work in different ways to induce sleep.

Benzodiazepines are sedative drugs that work by increasing the activity of the neurotransmitter GABA in the brain, which promotes feelings of relaxation and drowsiness. They are often prescribed to help reduce anxiety, relax muscles and induce sleep. Common examples of benzodiazepines include diazepam, lorazepam and alprazolam.

Zolpidem is a hypnotic drug that works more specifically on GABA receptors in the brain, helping to induce sleep. It is often used to treat short-term insomnia, helping to reduce the time it takes to fall asleep and improve sleep quality. Zolpidem is generally recommended for immediate use before bedtime and should not be used for long periods.

It is important to highlight that the use of sleeping pills should only be considered under proper medical guidance and prescription. These drugs can be effective in treating sleep disorders, but their use should be limited to specific situations and in the short term. The primary aim is to provide symptomatic relief while other therapeutic approaches such as cognitive behavioral therapy for insomnia (CBT-I) and lifestyle changes are implemented.

There are some important points to consider when using sleeping pills. First, these medications can cause side effects such as residual drowsiness during the day, dizziness, mental confusion, difficulty concentrating, and memory problems. Also, some individuals can develop a tolerance to the medications over time, meaning the dose needs to be increased to get the same effect. In rarer cases, dependence or abuse of these drugs can occur, especially if they are used inappropriately or for long periods.

For these reasons, it is essential to follow medical advice and use sleep medications with caution. They should be considered as a temporary option while pursuing more comprehensive therapeutic approaches such as behavioral therapy, lifestyle adjustments, and relaxation techniques. In addition, it is important to communicate regularly with your doctor to assess your continued need for these medications and to monitor any side effects or concerns about addiction.

## Possible consequences of using sleeping pills:

The use of sleeping pills can be associated with a number of consequences and side effects, and it is important to be aware of these aspects when considering this treatment option. Some common side effects include:

**Daytime sleepiness:**Sleeping medications can cause a feeling of residual drowsiness during the day, which can negatively affect concentration, memory, and the ability to carry out daily tasks.

**Memory and coordination difficulties:**Some sleep medications can interfere with cognitive function, resulting in memory difficulties, lack of mental clarity, and impaired motor coordination.

**Paradoxical sleep disorders:** In some cases, sleep medications can cause the opposite of the desired effects, resulting in paradoxical sleep disturbances. This can include agitation, nightmares, restlessness and worsened insomnia.

In addition to side effects, there are risks associated with long-term use or abuse of sleep medications. Some of these risks include:

**Dependency and Tolerance:**Continuous use of sleeping pills can lead to addiction, meaning the body becomes less responsive to the same dose, requiring higher doses to get the same effect. This can lead to a vicious cycle of increasing the dose and increasing dependency on the medications.

**rebound effect:** When sleep medications are stopped abruptly, a rebound effect can occur, resulting in worsened insomnia and difficulty sleeping. This is due to the body's adaptation to the effects of medications.

**Drug interactions:** Sleep medications can interact with other medications a person is taking, increasing the risk of side effects and complications.

It is critical to follow your doctor's advice when using sleep medications and to consider other options before resorting to them. Sleeping medications should only be used as a last resort and for short periods of time when other non-pharmacological approaches have not been effective. It is important to explore other treatment options, such as behavioral insomnia therapy (CBT-I), lifestyle changes, and relaxation techniques, which may be safer and more sustainable in the long term.

If the use of sleeping pills is necessary, it is essential to follow the prescribed dosages and medical guidelines, communicate regularly with the doctor about the effects and gradually adjust the dose, if necessary. Continuous monitoring is essential to prevent addiction, minimize associated risks and ensure a safe and effective treatment approach.

***

It is true that supplements and natural remedies can be considered as complementary options to promote healthy sleep. However, it is important to highlight that these products must be used with care and under proper guidance. While they may be effective for some people, it is essential to remember that each individual is unique and may respond differently to these supplements and natural remedies.

When considering the use of dietary supplements such as herbs, vitamins or minerals, it is essential to consult a qualified health professional such as a physician, nutritionist or herbalist. These professionals can assess your individual needs, medical history, and medications you are taking to guide you in choosing and dosing appropriate supplements.

Calming teas such as chamomile, valerian and lavender can be a natural option to promote relaxation and sleep. However, it is important to remember that, even though these teas are natural, they can have unwanted effects and drug interactions. It is recommended to seek guidance from a healthcare professional before including these teas in your sleep routine.

Likewise, essential oils such as lavender and chamomile can be used to promote relaxation and sleep. However, it is important to dilute oils correctly and follow proper usage guidelines. Also, some people may be sensitive to essential oils or have specific allergies, so it's important to perform a sensitivity test before applying them to large areas of the body. Guidance from a qualified aromatherapist can be helpful in understanding the correct dosage and application of essential oils.

It is crucial to point out that the misuse of any supplement or natural remedy can have risks and consequences. Some supplements may interact with medications you are taking or have unwanted side effects. Therefore, it is essential to seek medical advice before starting any treatment, even if it is natural.

In general, the safest and most effective approach is to take an integrative approach to improving sleep. This involves combining natural strategies such as teas, essential oils and supplements with lifestyle changes, relaxation techniques and proper sleep hygiene. When seeking complementary options, it is important to consider each person's individuality and work collaboratively with qualified healthcare professionals to find the best approach for your specific needs.

## Strategies for Different Stages of Life

*Tips for sleeping well during childhood, adolescence, adulthood and old age*

<u>Infancy</u>

During infancy, establishing a consistent sleep routine is critical to promoting healthy, developmentally appropriate sleep in children. From the first months of life, it is recommended to create a routine that includes regular sleep, wake up and bed times, helping to regulate the baby's biological clock.

In addition, it is important to create a calm and comfortable environment in the baby's room. This includes controlling the room temperature so that it is adequate, not too hot or too cold, providing comfort during sleep. It is also recommended to maintain a dark and silent environment, as darkness helps in the production of melatonin, the sleep hormone, while silence helps to minimize disturbances during sleep.

Encouraging the practice of relaxing activities before bed can also be beneficial for the child. Reading stories, singing lullabies, or taking a warm bath are examples of activities that help create a smooth transition to sleep. These practices help to calm the child and signal that it is time to relax and prepare for bed.

It is important to note that each child is unique and may have individual sleep needs. Also, routines may need to be adjusted as the child grows and goes through different stages of development. Observing the child's sleep signs and being aware of their needs is essential to establish a proper routine and ensure healthy sleep.

By promoting a consistent sleep routine, creating an environment conducive to rest, and encouraging relaxing activities before bed, parents are contributing to the establishment of good sleep habits from childhood. This not only helps the child get quality sleep, but also promotes their healthy development and overall well-being.

## Adolescence

During adolescence, it is important to establish regular sleep schedules, even on weekends. That means sticking to a consistent routine, going to bed and waking up at the same times every day, including free days. This practice helps to regulate the biological clock and improves the quality of sleep.

Also, limiting the use of electronic devices before bedtime is key. The blue light emitted by these devices can interfere with melatonin production, making it difficult to fall asleep. It is recommended to avoid using smartphones, tablets and computers at least one hour before bedtime. It is important to create an environment conducive to sleep, moving electronic devices away from the bedroom or using features such as the night mode, which reduces the emission of blue light.

Regular physical activity also plays an important role in promoting healthy sleep during adolescence. Physical exercise helps to regulate the circadian rhythm, promoting a feeling of physical fatigue that makes it easier to fall asleep. In addition, regular physical activity also helps reduce anxiety and stress, contributing to better sleep quality.

It is essential that teenagers understand the importance of sleep for their health and well-being. Hormones, growth, and physical and cognitive development occur primarily during sleep. Having adequate sleep contributes to academic performance, concentration, memory and emotional regulation.

By establishing regular sleep schedules, limiting electronic device use before bed, and encouraging regular physical activity, teens are creating healthy sleep habits that will benefit their health and well-being throughout their lives. It is important that they understand that these measures are essential to ensure a good quality of sleep and a better quality of life.

## adult life

In adult life, maintaining a regular sleep routine is essential to ensure a good quality of rest. Even with daily responsibilities and commitments, it's important to establish consistent sleep schedules, going to bed and waking up at the same times each day. This helps regulate the body clock and improves sleep efficiency.

Also, creating an environment conducive to sleep is essential. A comfortable mattress that offers adequate support to the body, a room with a pleasant and controlled temperature, noise reduction and minimization of light contribute to a peaceful and welcoming sleep environment. It is important to invest in a quality mattress that meets individual needs for comfort and firmness preference.

Practicing relaxation techniques before bed can also be beneficial for adults. Meditation, for example, can help reduce stress, anxiety and mental agitation, preparing the mind and body for sleep. Taking a few minutes before bed to meditate or practice deep breathing techniques can promote deep relaxation and a smooth transition to sleep.

Importantly, in adult life, sleep plays a crucial role in overall health and well-being. Having adequate sleep improves cognitive functioning, concentration capacity, decision making, in addition to strengthening the immune system and reducing the risk of chronic diseases. Therefore, it is essential to value sleep as an essential part of a healthy lifestyle.

By maintaining a regular sleep routine, creating an environment conducive to rest and practicing relaxation techniques, adults can optimize sleep quality and enjoy the benefits of a balanced and healthy life. These practices can improve energy, productivity and overall quality of life, allowing them to tackle daily challenges more effectively.

## Third Age

As you age, establishing a consistent sleep routine is especially important to promote healthy, restful sleep. This involves having regular bedtime and waking times, even on weekends, to help regulate your body clock and improve sleep quality.

In addition, engaging in regular physical activity during the day can be beneficial in promoting healthy tiredness at night. Exercises such as walking, yoga or swimming help improve sleep quality, stimulate blood circulation and reduce stress. However, it is important to avoid intense activities too close to bedtime, as this can make it difficult to relax and transition to sleep.

Old age often involves the use of medication to treat chronic medical conditions. Some medications can affect sleep, causing insomnia or excessive sleepiness. It is important to talk to your doctor about the medications you are taking and discuss the possibility of adjustments in dosage or time of administration to minimize negative effects on sleep. The doctor will be able to assess which changes are appropriate, considering the individual's general health.

In addition, it is important to ensure a conducive sleep environment. This includes having a comfortable mattress, controlling the temperature in the room, reducing noise and blocking out excessive light. Creating a peaceful, pleasant bedroom environment can help promote more restful, restful sleep.

Valuing sleep in old age is essential to promote a good quality of life. Adequate sleep contributes to physical and mental health, improves memory, concentration and disposition during the day. By establishing a consistent sleep routine, practicing regular physical activity and monitoring the medications being used, seniors can optimize their sleep quality and enjoy a healthier and more balanced life.

*Sleep during pregnancy and the necessary care for mothers-to-be*

## Sleep care during pregnancy

During pregnancy, many women face sleep challenges due to a number of physical and hormonal factors. As your pregnancy progresses, physical discomfort such as back pain, an enlarged belly, and difficulty finding a comfortable sleeping position can affect your sleep quality. Additionally, hormonal changes can cause changes in sleep patterns, leading to feeling constantly tired or having difficulty falling asleep.

However, there are some strategies that can help improve sleep during pregnancy. One of them is to use pillows for support. Pillows can be positioned between the legs to relieve pressure on the hips and lower back, or they can be used to support the belly and provide greater comfort when sleeping on your side, which is the recommended position for pregnant women.

Maintaining good sleep hygiene is also important during pregnancy. This includes maintaining an environment conducive to sleep, with a comfortable mattress, temperature control and noise and light reduction. Additionally, establishing a relaxing bedtime routine, such as taking a warm bath, practicing relaxation techniques, or reading a book, can help prepare your body and mind for a good night's sleep.

Adopting comfortable sleeping positions is also key. During pregnancy, sleeping on your side, preferably the left side, can help improve blood flow to your baby and relieve pressure on internal organs. Using pillows to support your back, belly, and legs can help you find a more comfortable position.

It is essential to experiment with different techniques and strategies to discover what provides the best comfort and quality of sleep during pregnancy. If the difficulties persist or sleep continues to be a challenge, it is recommended to talk to the obstetrician, who will be able to offer personalized and appropriate guidance for each specific case.

## Preparation for sleep after childbirth

After the baby is born, the mother's sleep patterns can be challenging due to the newborn's needs, such as nighttime breastfeeding and irregular sleep cycles. It is important to remember that babies have a constant need for food, comfort and attention, which can interfere with the quantity and quality of the mother's sleep.

One of the suggestions for dealing with these challenges is to establish a sleep routine for the baby. This can include setting regular bedtime and waking times, creating a peaceful environment conducive to sleep, such as a dark, quiet room, and using relaxation techniques, such as snuggling the baby and calming the atmosphere before putting her to sleep. Following a consistent routine can help your baby feel secure and comfortable, as well as ease the transition to sleep.

Sharing nighttime responsibilities with your partner can also be an effective strategy. This allows both parents the opportunity to rest and take turns in caring for the baby during the night. With a collaborative approach, you can share your baby's sleep demands and ensure that both of you have a chance to regain your energy.

Seeking moments of rest during the day is also important for the mother. Taking advantage of the moments when the baby is sleeping to rest or take naps can help compensate for nighttime sleep deprivation. It is essential that the mother takes care of her own health and well-being, prioritizing rest whenever possible.

It is important to remember that sleep after childbirth can be fragmented and disrupted. This is part of the process of adapting to the new routine with the baby. As the baby grows and develops more regular sleep patterns, the mother will have the opportunity to gradually regain her normal sleep. Patience and understanding are key in this transition period.

Each mother and baby is unique, and it is important to seek appropriate support and guidance during this time. Talking to other parents, joining support groups, and seeking advice from healthcare professionals who specialize in childcare can offer valuable support and tips for dealing with postpartum sleep challenges.

*** 

Recognizing and addressing specific sleep challenges at different stages of life is essential to promoting healthy sleep at all stages. Each phase of life has unique characteristics that can affect the quantity and quality of sleep, and it is important to adopt strategies adapted to each one of them.

During childhood, establishing a consistent sleep routine from the first few months is essential. This involves creating a peaceful and comfortable environment in the baby's room, with adequate temperature and light control. Also, engaging in relaxing activities before bed, such as stories or warm baths, can help prepare your baby for sleep.

In adolescence, when sleep patterns undergo significant changes, it is important to establish regular sleep schedules, even during weekends. Limiting the use of electronic devices before bedtime is also crucial due to the stimulating effects of blue light. Regular practice of physical activities during the day can help regulate the circadian rhythm and reduce anxiety, contributing to healthier sleep.

During adult life, maintaining a regular sleep routine is essential, even with daily commitments and responsibilities. Creating an environment conducive to sleep, with a comfortable mattress, adequate temperature control and reduction of noise and light, is important to promote quality sleep. Additionally, practicing relaxation techniques such as meditation before bed can help reduce stress and promote relaxation.

In old age, establishing a consistent sleep routine is also essential. Regular physical activity during the day can promote healthy tiredness at night, helping to improve sleep quality. It is important to monitor medications that may affect sleep and discuss adjustments in dosage or time of administration with the physician, taking into account possible drug interactions.

It is essential to highlight that, at any stage of life, it is important to seek medical advice when specific sleep problems arise. A specialist healthcare professional will be able to assess the situation on an individual basis, consider health and lifestyle factors, and offer appropriate guidance and treatments to promote healthy sleep.

In summary, addressing the specific sleep challenges at each stage of life is essential to promoting healthy sleep and improving quality of life. By adopting strategies adapted to each phase and seeking medical advice when necessary, it is possible to face sleep challenges effectively and enjoy the benefits of restful sleep at all stages of life.

# Managing Jet Lag and Irregular Timings

*Tips for minimizing the effects of jet lag after travel*

Entendendo o jet lag

Jet lag is a condition that occurs when traveling to regions with different time zones, affecting our internal body clock, also known as circadian rhythm. The circadian rhythm is responsible for regulating sleep-wake cycles, body temperature and other biological processes.

When we cross time zones, our body needs to adapt to a new local time, which can take some time. During this adaptation process, it is common to experience jet lag symptoms. These symptoms can vary from person to person, but the most common ones include fatigue, daytime sleepiness, difficulty sleeping, irritability, problems concentrating, changes in appetite and headaches.

The main reason why jet lag occurs is because our circadian rhythm is synchronized with the time we are used to sleeping and waking up. When we cross time zones, this synchronization is interrupted and it takes some time for our body to adjust to the new local time. The mismatch between the body's internal time and local time is what causes jet lag symptoms.

There are some strategies that can help minimize the effects of jet lag and make it easier to adapt to the new local time. It is recommended to gradually adjust your sleep schedule a few days before travel, trying to adapt to the local time at the destination. During the flight, it is important to stay hydrated, avoid excessive consumption of alcohol and caffeine, and try to rest or sleep according to the new local time. Upon arrival at your destination, it is recommended to expose yourself to natural light during the day and avoid exposure to bright light before bed to help readjust your circadian rhythm.

In some cases, medication or light therapy may be needed to help adjust the circadian rhythm more quickly. However, it is important to consult a healthcare professional before taking any medication or starting any therapy to treat jet lag.

In summary, jet lag is a common effect of traveling across time zones, causing circadian rhythm disruption and resulting in symptoms such as fatigue, difficulty sleeping and irritability. Adopting appropriate strategies, such as gradually adjusting your sleep schedule before travel, exposing yourself to natural light during the day, and avoiding exposure to bright light before bed, can help minimize the effects of jet lag and make it easier to adapt to the new environment. local time.

## Preparation before the trip

Proper pre-travel preparation plays an important role in minimizing the effects of jet lag. Here are some suggestions to prepare for your trip:

**Gradual adjustment of sleep schedule:** A few days before your trip, try to gradually adjust your sleep schedule according to your destination. If you're traveling east, try to sleep a little earlier. If traveling west, try to sleep a little later. This gradual change helps the body adapt to the new schedule.

**Adjusting meal times:** As with sleep, try to gradually adjust your meal times according to your destination. This includes main meals as well as snacks. Eating according to local time can help synchronize your body's rhythm with the new time zone.

**Proper hydration:** Dehydration can exacerbate the effects of jet lag, so it's important to stay well hydrated before and during your flight. Drink water regularly and avoid excessive consumption of alcohol, caffeine and sugary drinks, which can dehydrate the body. Remember that air humidity inside the airplane cabin tends to be low, so it's important to compensate for this moisture loss by drinking adequate water.

**Avoid overindulging in meals:** Before the flight, avoid heavy or high-fat meals, which can cause discomfort and make it difficult to sleep during the flight. Opt for light, balanced meals that are easy to digest. Also, avoid eating too close to bedtime, as this can interfere with the quality of sleep during the flight.

**Avoid sudden changes in sleep schedule:** In the days leading up to the trip, avoid sudden big changes in your sleep schedule. This can further disrupt your circadian rhythm. Try to maintain a consistent and regular sleep routine to help your body adapt more smoothly to the new schedule.

By following these suggestions before your trip, you will help your body gradually adjust to the new time zone. This can make it easier to adapt to your destination and reduce the negative effects of jet lag, allowing you to better enjoy your trip and adapt more quickly to the new local time.

## During flight

While flying, there are a few strategies you can adopt to help minimize the effects of jet lag. Here are some recommendations for adjusting to the new time zone while flying:

**Clock settings:** Once the plane takes off, set your clocks to the destination time. This helps mentally synchronize your body with the new time zone and prepare for the transition.

**Stay hydrated:** Drinking water regularly during the flight is key to staying hydrated. Low air humidity in the airplane cabin can lead to dehydration, which can worsen jet lag symptoms. Avoid alcohol and caffeine, as these substances can interfere with sleep quality and increase dehydration.

**Move around and do light exercise:** During the flight, it is important to move regularly and do light exercises to stimulate blood circulation and prevent muscle stiffness. Get up and walk down the aisle of the plane whenever possible. Additionally, you can perform stretching exercises in your seat to ease muscle tension and promote blood flow.

**Avoid long naps:** If you're flying during the day, avoid long naps, as this can make it difficult to adjust to the new time zone. Try to stay awake and enjoy natural light inside the plane, especially if you're traveling east. If you need to rest, opt for short, planned naps.

**Exposure to light:** Light exposure has a significant impact on the circadian rhythm. During the flight, adjust the blinds to let in natural light or use a sleep mask to block out the light, depending on your purpose. If you are flying during the day to a night time destination, try to avoid excessive exposure to bright light. On the other hand, if you're flying at night to a daytime destination, try to expose yourself to natural light as soon as possible.

## upon arrival

Upon arrival at your destination, some strategies can be adopted to help adjust the internal clock to the new time zone and minimize the effects of jet lag. Here are some suggestions:

**Exposure to natural light:** Exposing yourself to natural light during the day is one of the best ways to help synchronize your internal clock with the new local time. Spend time outside, especially in the early hours of the morning, to help suppress melatonin production (the sleep hormone) and signal your body that it's time to be awake. Avoid wearing sunglasses during this time to allow natural light to enter your eyes.

**Avoid exposure to artificial light at night:** Exposure to artificial light at night can interfere with melatonin production and make it difficult to sleep. Reduce exposure to blue light emitted by electronic devices, such as smartphones and tablets, a few hours before bed. Also, use curtains or blinds to block outside light into the bedroom at night, creating a dark, sleep-friendly environment.

**Immediate adjustment of meals and activities:** Try to adapt to your local meal and activity schedule as quickly as possible, even if that means fighting drowsiness during the day. This will help realign your circadian rhythm with the new schedule. Avoid eating heavy meals late at night, as this can make it difficult for your digestive system and sleep to adjust to the new time zone.

**Strategic naps:** If you are experiencing excessive sleepiness during the day, it may be helpful to take short, strategic naps to help combat fatigue. Naps of 20 to 30 minutes can provide an energy boost without interfering with nighttime sleep. Avoid long naps, as they can impair your ability to sleep at night.

**Regular physical activity:** Regular exercise can help regulate your circadian rhythm and promote feelings of alertness throughout the day. Do moderate-intensity physical activity during the day to help boost energy and reduce drowsiness.

Adapting to the new time zone can take a few days, and everyone reacts differently. The key is to be consistent with the adjustment strategies and allow your body to gradually adapt to the new schedule. If you continue to experience significant difficulties with jet lag, it may be helpful to seek medical advice for additional advice and support.

## *Strategies for people who work shifts or have irregular sleep schedules*

### Understanding the challenges of irregular hours

Night, shift, or irregular work schedules can present significant challenges to sleep quality and quantity. Here are some aspects to consider:

**Disruption of circadian rhythm:** The circadian rhythm is the body's internal clock that regulates sleep and waking patterns. Shift or night work can disrupt this natural rhythm, as you are working when the body would normally be resting. This can lead to a constant struggle to adjust your internal clock and make it difficult to get adequate sleep.

**I'm fragmented:** Irregular work schedules can lead to fragmented sleep, as you may need to sleep during the day when light and noise are most intense. In addition, the need to adapt to different work schedules can cause your sleep to be interrupted regularly, affecting the quality of rest.

**Fatigue and daytime sleepiness:** Lack of adequate sleep due to irregular working hours can lead to fatigue and excessive daytime sleepiness. This can negatively affect productivity, concentration and performance at work, as well as increase the risk of accidents.

**Impact on physical and mental health:** Chronic sleep deprivation due to irregular working hours can have negative consequences for physical and mental health. It can increase the risk of developing cardiovascular disease, diabetes, obesity, and mental health disorders such as anxiety and depression. Additionally, disruption of the circadian rhythm can lead to digestive, metabolic, and hormonal issues.

**Difficulties in reconciling work and personal life:** Irregular working hours can jeopardize the balance between work and personal life. Lack of adequate sleep can affect relationships, participation in social activities and family involvement, as well as limit the time available for rest and self-care.

Faced with these challenges, it is important to adopt strategies to minimize the negative impacts of irregular working hours on sleep and health. Some suggestions include:

**Establish a consistent routine:** Try to keep regular sleep schedules, even if they differ from your traditional schedule. Establish a routine that allows enough time for rest and recovery.

**Create an environment conducive to sleep:** Use techniques to create a dark, quiet, and comfortable sleeping environment, no matter what time you need to rest. Use sleep masks, earplugs and blackout curtains to help block out outside light and noise.

**Practice proper sleep hygiene:** Adopt healthy sleep habits, such as avoiding the consumption of stimulants before bed, maintaining a cool and suitable environment for sleep, and avoiding the use of electronic devices before bed.

**Prioritize self-care:** Find time for relaxing and self-care activities, such as regular exercise, relaxation techniques, hobbies, and leisure time. This can help reduce stress and promote more restful sleep.

**Seek professional support:** If you are experiencing significant difficulties with irregular work schedules and sleep, it is recommended that you seek medical advice or consult a specialist in sleep disorders. They can provide personalized guidance and specific strategies for dealing with sleep challenges in this context.

## Managing irregular hours

Managing irregular work schedules can be challenging, but there are strategies that can help minimize sleep impacts and promote adequate rest. Here are some approaches to managing irregular hours:

**Establish a consistent routine:** Even with variable work schedules, try to create a consistent sleep schedule, keeping regular bedtimes and waking times whenever possible. This helps train your body and regulate your internal clock, making it easier to fall asleep and wake up, regardless of the time.

**Create an environment conducive to sleep:** Regardless of what time you need to sleep, create a suitable environment to promote sleep. This includes having a room that is dark, quiet and cool, regardless of the time of day. Use blackout curtains, ear plugs and adjust the room temperature to make the room as comfortable as possible.

**Use relaxation techniques:** Regardless of what time you need to sleep, it's important to adopt relaxation techniques to calm your mind and body before bed. This can include practices such as meditation, deep breathing, guided visualizations or progressive muscle relaxation techniques. These techniques help reduce stress and prepare the body for sleep, regardless of the time of day.

**Manage exposure to light:** Light exposure plays a crucial role in regulating the circadian rhythm. During waking hours, aim for exposure to natural light as much as possible. This helps keep your internal clock set and promotes vigilance while working. Before bed, avoid excessive exposure to bright light, especially from electronic devices, as blue light can interfere with the production of melatonin, the sleep hormone.

**Plan adequate rest periods:** If your work schedules are irregular, it's important to plan adequate rest periods between shifts. Be sure to allow enough time to rest and regain energy before starting your next shift. This could involve short naps or strategic rest periods throughout the day.

**Communicating your needs to co-workers:** If possible, communicate your sleep needs and ask coworkers for cooperation. Explain the importance of having a quiet environment during rest and ask for support to minimize noise and unnecessary interruptions.

**Prioritize self-care:** Managing irregular schedules requires careful attention to self-care. Make sure you prioritize eating healthy, exercising regularly, and making time for relaxing activities. These practices contribute to overall health and help promote better quality sleep.

## Health care

Taking care of your health is key, especially when dealing with irregular work schedules. Here are some important points to consider:

**Balanced and healthy diet:** Even with irregular schedules, it's essential to provide your body with the nutrients it needs to keep you healthy and energized. Prioritize nutritious foods like fruits, vegetables, lean proteins and whole grains. Avoid processed and high-sugar foods, as they can negatively affect sleep and overall health. Plan your meals in advance and opt for quick, healthy options like salads, sandwiches or pre-prepared meals at home.

**Practice of regular physical activity:** Even with irregular schedules, finding time to exercise is key to promoting quality sleep and overall well-being. Regular physical activity helps reduce stress, improve mood and increase energy levels. Find activities that you enjoy and that fit into your routine, such as walking, jogging, dancing classes, or exercising at home. Even small exercise sessions can have a significant positive impact on your health.

**Stress management and emotional care:** Irregular work schedules can cause stress and emotional challenges. It's important to look for healthy ways to deal with stress, such as relaxation techniques, meditation, yoga or therapy. Find activities that help you relax and de-stress, such as listening to music, reading a book, pursuing hobbies, or spending time with loved ones. If emotional challenges persist, do not hesitate to seek professional support from a psychologist or therapist, who can help you develop effective coping strategies.

**Adequate sleep:** Even with irregular schedules, prioritizing adequate sleep is essential. Establish a consistent sleep routine whenever possible by creating an environment conducive to sleep, maintaining a comfortable bedroom temperature, and avoiding distracting stimuli before bed. If necessary, consider using relaxation techniques or meditation to help calm your mind and facilitate sleep. If sleep problems persist, it is recommended to seek medical advice to identify and treat possible sleep disorders.

**General health care:** In addition to the aspects mentioned above, it is important to keep regular medical appointments and take care of your health comprehensively. Get routine checkups, monitor your blood pressure, control your weight, and take care of any existing medical conditions. Stay up to date with recommended vaccinations and follow your doctor's guidelines to ensure overall good health.

## How to adjust the internal clock and maintain consistency even under challenging circumstances

### Adjusting the internal clock

Adjusting the body's internal clock is essential for improving sleep quality and promoting a healthy routine. Here is some information and suggestions to help with this process:

**circadian rhythm:** The circadian rhythm is an approximately 24-hour biological cycle that regulates the body's physiological processes, including sleep and wakefulness. Strengthening the circadian rhythm is key to establishing a regular sleep and waking pattern. The body has a natural ability to adapt to regular sleep and wake times, and this can be achieved by creating a consistent routine.

**Exposure to natural light during the day:** Natural light is one of the main stimuli to regulate the circadian rhythm. By exposing yourself to natural light first thing in the morning, you are telling your body that it is time to wake up and start your day. Open the blinds, go for a walk or have breakfast next to a window to take advantage of the natural light. This will help suppress the production of melatonin, the sleep hormone, and help set your internal clock to be alert during the day.

**Darkness at night:** As the day draws to a close, it's important to create a dark environment to help prepare the body for sleep. This means reducing exposure to artificial light, especially the blue light emitted by electronic devices, before bed. Turn off electronic devices, use blackout curtains or sleep shades to block outside light, and create a dark, peaceful bedroom environment. Darkness signals the brain that it's time to produce melatonin and start the sleep process.

**Maintain regular schedules:** Establishing regular sleep and wake times is key to synchronizing the body's internal clock. Try to go to bed and wake up at approximately the same time each day, including weekends. This helps to strengthen the circadian rhythm and regulate the body's biological processes.

**Avoid disturbing stimuli before sleeping:** In addition to controlling exposure to light, it is important to avoid stimuli that may interfere with sleep quality. Avoid caffeine consumption, heavy food and stimulating activities before bed. Try to adopt relaxation rituals, such as taking a warm bath, reading a book or practicing breathing techniques, to help prepare your body and mind for sleep.

The important thing is to find a balance that works for you and your routine. If sleep problems persist or if you have significant difficulties adjusting your internal clock, it is recommended that you seek medical advice to identify and treat possible sleep disorders or obtain specific guidance for your case.

Adjusting your internal clock can take time and patience, but with consistency and healthy practices, you can help your body regulate sleep more effectively and improve the quality of your rest.

## Additional Strategies

In addition to the previously mentioned strategies, there are other approaches that can be helpful in adjusting sleep, especially during challenging times. Here are some additional strategies:

**Relaxation techniques:** Meditation and breathing exercises are effective practices for calming the mind and relaxing the body, easing the transition to sleep. Meditation involves focusing attention on the present moment, letting go of intrusive thoughts and worries. Regular meditation practice can help reduce anxiety and stress, promoting a state of calm and tranquility before bed. In addition, breathing exercises such as deep abdominal breathing can activate the parasympathetic nervous system, which is responsible for the body's relaxation response.

**Avoid caffeine and stimulants:** Caffeine is a known stimulant that can interfere with sleep. Avoid caffeine consumption, including coffee, black tea, soft drinks and chocolate, especially around bedtime. In addition to caffeine, be aware of other stimulants such as tobacco and certain medications that can affect sleep quality. Opt for decaffeinated beverages and choose more relaxing alternatives like herbal teas or water, especially at night.

**Manage sleep environment:** Create an environment conducive to sleep, no matter what time you sleep. This includes keeping the room cool, dark, and quiet. Use blackout curtains or sleep shades to block out excessive light, use earplugs or white noise machines to minimize distracting noises, and make sure your mattress and pillow offer adequate support and comfort.

**Establish a relaxation routine:** Take time to relax and wind down before bed, regardless of the time of day. This could include activities such as taking a warm bath, reading a calming book, listening to soft music, or doing gentle stretches. These practices help prepare the body and mind for sleep, signaling the nervous system that it is time to relax and rest.

By adopting these additional strategies, you will be strengthening the favorable conditions for more restful and revitalizing sleep, even at challenging times. Consistency and the incorporation of healthy sleep habits can significantly contribute to improving the quality of your rest and, consequently, to your overall well-being.

***

Living amid challenges like jet lag and irregular sleep schedules can certainly impact the quality and consistency of our sleep. However, it is important to highlight that there are effective strategies to manage these situations and promote healthy sleep, even in challenging circumstances.

In the case of jet lag, which occurs when traveling across different time zones, it is essential to adopt measures that help adapt our circadian rhythm to the new local time. Here are some tips for minimizing the effects of jet lag:

**gradual adjustment:** Before traveling, try to gradually adjust your sleeping and eating schedule according to where you are going. This may involve bringing forward or delaying bedtime and waking up a few days before travel, depending on the destination time zone.

**Proper hydration:** During the flight, it's important to stay hydrated, as dehydration can exacerbate the effects of jet lag. Drink water regularly and avoid excessive consumption of alcohol, caffeine and sugary drinks, which can interfere with sleep and adequate hydration.

**Immediate adjustment to local time:** As soon as you arrive at your destination, immediately adjust your clocks to the local time zone. Try to expose yourself to natural light during the day, as this will help regulate your internal clock. Avoid napping for long periods of time during the day and stick to local times for meals and activities.

Regarding irregular sleep schedules, such as working at night, in shifts or at alternate times, it is essential to adopt measures that minimize the negative impacts on sleep quality and general well-being. Here are some strategies that can help:

**Create a consistent routine:** Even with variable work schedules, it's important to establish a regular sleep routine. Try to go to sleep and wake up at approximately the same times every day, even on your days off. This will help regulate your circadian rhythm and promote more consistent sleep.

**Manage sleep environment:**Regardless of what time you sleep, create an environment conducive to sleep. Make sure your bedroom is cool, dark and quiet. Use blackout curtains or sleep shades to block out excessive light, use ear plugs or white noise machines to minimize distracting noise, and choose a comfortable mattress and pillows that suit your preferences.

**Adapt the light exposure:**Exposure to light is an important factor in regulating the circadian rhythm. If you work overnight, avoid exposure to bright sunlight on your way home, as this can throw off your internal clock. During the day, try to expose yourself to natural light as much as possible, either by taking a walk outside or leaving the curtains open. During the night, reduce exposure to artificial light, especially near bedtime, to help signal your body that it's time to rest.

**Create an environment conducive to sleep:** Regardless of what time you sleep, it's important to follow a relaxing bedtime routine. Avoid using electronic devices before bed, as the blue light emitted by them can interfere with the production of melatonin, a hormone that regulates sleep. Instead, opt for relaxing activities like reading a book, taking a warm bath, or practicing relaxation techniques like meditation or deep breathing.

In summary, although jet lag and irregular sleep schedules can present challenges to healthy sleep, it is possible to minimize their effects by adopting specific strategies. Consistency in the sleep routine, care for the resting environment, adequate exposure to natural light and the practice of relaxing habits are essential to adjust the internal clock and promote quality sleep, regardless of challenging circumstances.

# I am and Saude Mental

*The link between sleep and mental health: How sleep deprivation can affect mood, anxiety and depression*

<u>Importance of sleep for mental health</u>

Sleep plays a key role in mental health, and the relationship between them is two-way. Getting adequate sleep is essential to promoting good mental health, while poor mental health can negatively affect the quality and duration of sleep.

Sleep deprivation can have significant impacts on mood regulation, anxiety and depression. When we don't get enough sleep, it's common to experience irritability, mood swings and concentration difficulties. In addition, lack of adequate sleep can increase sensitivity to stress, making it more difficult to deal with everyday challenges.

The relationship between sleep and mental health is especially evident in anxiety and depression. Lack of sleep can increase anxiety and contribute to feelings of constant worry. On the other hand, anxiety can also interfere with the ability to fall asleep and maintain restful sleep.

Likewise, chronic sleep deprivation is associated with a higher risk of developing and recurring depressive symptoms. Lack of sleep affects neurotransmitters and brain processes involved in mood regulation, which can contribute to the development and worsening of depression.

Adequate sleep plays a vital role in memory consolidation and emotional processing. During sleep, the brain consolidates the information learned during the day, facilitating memory and learning. It is also during sleep that we process and regulate emotions, which is essential for mental health and the ability to deal with stressful situations.

It is therefore crucial to recognize the importance of sleep for mental health and take steps to ensure adequate sleep. This includes adopting a regular sleep routine, creating an environment conducive to sleep, practicing relaxation techniques before bed, and seeking medical help if there are persistent difficulties with sleep or mental health issues.

By prioritizing sleep and taking care of mental health, it is possible to improve general well-being, increase emotional resilience and have a better quality of life. Adequate sleep and mental health are intertwined, and investing in both is key to promoting a healthy and balanced life.

## Impact of sleep deprivation on mental health

Sleep deprivation has a significant impact on mental health, affecting the regulation of emotions and the ability to cope with stress. When we don't get enough sleep, our nervous system is deregulated, making us more sensitive to everyday stressful and challenging situations.

One of the most obvious effects of sleep deprivation is the difficulty in emotional regulation. Sleeping little or having a compromised quality of sleep can lead to changes in the balance of neurotransmitters in the brain, affecting emotional stability. This can result in increased irritability, emotional lability, increased emotional reactivity, and difficulty controlling emotions.

In addition, chronic sleep deprivation is associated with a higher risk of developing mental disorders such as anxiety and depression. Studies show that people who sleep less than necessary are more likely to develop these disorders. The relationship between sleep and mental health is complex, but lack of sleep is believed to affect neurotransmitter systems and brain processes involved in mood regulation.

Anxiety and sleep deprivation are closely related. Lack of adequate sleep can increase anxiety and worry, making it harder to deal with daily challenges. In turn, anxiety can also make it difficult to fall asleep and maintain restful sleep.

In the case of depression, sleep deprivation can contribute to the development and worsening of symptoms. People with chronic sleep deprivation are more likely to develop depression and experience recurrence of symptoms after treatment. Lack of sleep affects the regulation of neurotransmitters such as serotonin, which plays a key role in regulating mood and feelings of well-being.

Additionally, sleep deprivation impairs cognitive function, which can negatively affect the ability to process information, make decisions, and solve problems. This can increase feelings of stress and mental overload, contributing to deteriorating mental health.

Sleep deprivation has a significant impact on mental health, increasing the risk of mental disorders, affecting emotional regulation and making it difficult to cope with stress. It is essential to recognize the importance of adequate sleep for mental health and to seek strategies to improve the quality and quantity of sleep, including adopting a consistent sleep routine, creating an environment conducive to sleeping and seeking professional help, when necessary.

## cycle of mutual influence

The relationship between sleep and mental health is characterized by a cycle of mutual influence, where mental health can affect sleep quality and, in turn, sleep quality can influence mental health. This two-way connection highlights the importance of addressing both mental health and sleep in an integrated way.

When it comes to the influence of mental health on sleep quality, it is important to highlight that mental disorders can directly affect sleep. For example, anxiety, depression, and chronic stress can cause difficulty falling asleep, staying asleep, or resulting in unrefreshing sleep. These disorders can lead to intrusive thoughts, constant worrying and overactive brain activity, making it difficult to relax and fall asleep. In addition, the neurochemical changes associated with these disorders can negatively affect circadian rhythms, impairing sleep regulation.

On the other hand, sleep quality also plays a key role in mental health. Sleep deprivation or poor sleep quality can negatively affect cognitive, emotional and behavioral functioning, increasing vulnerability to mental health problems. Lack of adequate sleep can lead to increased stress, irritability, difficulty concentrating, decreased motivation, and worsening symptoms of anxiety and depression.

There are neurobiological mechanisms involved in this relationship between sleep and mental health. Adequate sleep plays a crucial role in regulating neurotransmitters and hormones involved in mental health, such as serotonin, dopamine, noradrenaline and the stress hormone cortisol. Lack of sleep affects these neurochemical systems, impairing emotional stability, mood regulation and stress response.

In addition, lack of sleep interferes with memory consolidation processes and cognitive functioning, negatively affecting the ability to process information, make decisions and solve problems. This can contribute to feelings of hopelessness, low self-esteem and difficulty finding solutions to everyday challenges, which can affect mental health.

It is essential to address both mental health and sleep in an integrated way, recognizing the mutual influence between them. By taking care of mental health, seeking appropriate treatment for mental disorders and adopting strategies to manage stress and worries, it is possible to improve the quality of sleep. Likewise, prioritizing healthy sleep, adopting adequate sleep habits and seeking treatment for sleep problems can contribute to improved mental health.

## Strategies to improve sleep in cases of mental disorders

### Identifying and treating comorbid sleep disorders

The presence of comorbid sleep disorders, that is, sleep disorders that occur simultaneously with mental disorders, is a very common occurrence. Mental disorders such as anxiety, depression, bipolar disorder and post-traumatic stress disorders can be associated with a variety of sleep disorders.

Insomnia is one of the most common sleep disorders in individuals with mental disorders. People with anxiety, for example, may have difficulty relaxing and falling asleep due to intrusive thoughts and constant worrying. Likewise, people with depression may experience insomnia, which is characterized by difficulty falling asleep, waking up early, or fragmented, unrefreshing sleep.

Another common comorbid sleep disorder is sleep apnea, which occurs when breathing stops during sleep. Sleep apnea has been linked to a higher risk of mood disorders such as depression and bipolar disorder. In addition, sleep apnea can exacerbate symptoms of pre-existing mental disorders, contributing to fatigue, irritability and decreased quality of life.

Restless legs syndrome (RLS) is another comorbid sleep disorder that can affect mental health. RLS is characterized by an uncomfortable feeling in the legs, often accompanied by an overwhelming urge to move them. These symptoms can make it difficult to sleep and contribute to insomnia and irritability, negatively affecting mental well-being.

Identifying and treating these comorbid sleep disorders is essential for a comprehensive and effective approach to mental health care.

When sleep disorders are not treated in conjunction with mental disorders, there can be worsening of mental symptoms, difficulty responding to appropriate treatment, and a lower overall quality of life.

Treatment of these comorbid sleep disorders usually involves a multidisciplinary approach, which may include mental health professionals, sleep medicine specialists, and other health professionals. Depending on the type and severity of the sleep disorder, treatment options may include behavioral therapy such as cognitive behavioral therapy for insomnia, medical devices such as CPAP for apnea of sleep, specific medications or a combination of different approaches.

By addressing comorbid sleep disorders in conjunction with treating the underlying mental health, it is possible to improve sleep quality and reduce symptoms of mental disorders. Early identification and proper treatment of these sleep disorders can be key to promoting general well-being and improving the quality of life of those affected.

## Adapted sleep hygiene practices

Implementing adapted sleep hygiene practices is particularly important for people with mental disorders, as these conditions can negatively affect sleep and the quality of rest. The following are some specific sleep hygiene guidelines that may be helpful for individuals with mental disorders:

**Establish a consistent routine:** Having a regular sleep routine, going to bed and waking up at the same times each day, can help regulate your body's internal clock and improve sleep quality. It is recommended to maintain this routine, even on weekends.

**Create an environment conducive to sleep:** Create a quiet, comfortable and dark sleeping environment in the bedroom. Use blackout curtains or sleep shades to block out excessive light and reduce outside noise, such as using ear plugs or white noise machines. Ensure that the room temperature is adequate, cool and well ventilated.

**Manage stress and anxiety before bed:**People with mental disorders often experience high levels of stress and anxiety, which can make it difficult for them to sleep. Relaxation practices such as meditation, deep breathing, stretching exercises or yoga can help calm the mind and reduce tension before bed. Avoid stimulating activities, such as using electronic devices or watching emotionally charged programs, before bed.

**Avoid substances that interfere with sleep:**Certain substances can interfere with sleep and worsen the symptoms of mental disorders. It is recommended to avoid the consumption of caffeine, nicotine and alcohol before bed, as they can negatively affect the quality of sleep. Consult a healthcare professional for specific guidance on the relationship between medications used to treat mental disorders and sleep.

**Seek professional support:** It is important to seek help from health professionals, such as doctors, psychiatrists or psychologists, for the proper treatment of mental disorders and to receive specific guidance related to sleep. These professionals can assess the situation individually and offer personalized recommendations.

## Cognitive behavioral therapy for insomnia (CBT-I)

Cognitive-Behavioral Therapy for Insomnia (CBT-I) is a widely recognized and effective therapeutic approach in the treatment of chronic insomnia. It is based on principles of cognitive and behavioral psychology, aiming to identify and modify the thought patterns and behaviors that contribute to the maintenance of insomnia.

CBT-I is a structured form of therapy that involves collaboration between therapist and patient. The main objective is to re-educate sleep, helping the patient to develop healthy habits and behaviors in relation to sleep, and to modify negative thought patterns or concerns related to sleep.

CBT-I is made up of several components that address different aspects of insomnia. Some of the main components include:

**Sleep retraining:** This component involves identifying and modifying inappropriate sleep beliefs and behaviors. The therapist helps the patient establish a regular sleep routine, with consistent bedtime and wake-up times. Issues such as the importance of a suitable sleep environment and limiting stimulating activities before bedtime are also addressed.

**Relaxation techniques:** CBT-I includes teaching relaxation techniques such as deep breathing, meditation or progressive muscle relaxation. These techniques help reduce anxiety and muscle tension, making it easier to fall asleep.

**Stimulus Control:** Stimulus control involves establishing a positive association between the bedroom and sleep. This means limiting activities done in bed to just sleep and intimacy, and avoiding stimulating activities like watching TV or using electronic devices. This practice helps to strengthen the association between the bedroom and sleep, making the environment conducive to sleep.

**Sleep restriction:** Sleep restriction involves limiting the time the patient spends in bed to match the actual amount of sleep they are getting. This technique helps to consolidate sleep and reduce the time spent in bed without sleep. Over time, time in bed is gradually increased as sleep efficiency improves.

In addition to these core components, CBT-I can include other tailored strategies depending on the patient's individual needs. Therapy is usually carried out in a structured format, with regular sessions with a specialist sleep therapist.

CBT-I is considered a first-line treatment approach for chronic insomnia and has been proven to be effective in both the short and long term. It offers a safe and effective alternative to sleeping pills, especially for those who prefer non-pharmacological approaches or who have concerns about side effects. However, it's important to seek out a health professional who specializes in sleep or a cognitive-behavioral therapist to receive specific guidance and a personalized treatment plan.

## Complementary therapies to promote mental health through sleep

### Sono therapy and complementary therapies:

Complementary therapies such as acupuncture, chiropractic and music therapy are increasingly being explored as treatment options for sleep disorders and mental health issues. Although research in this field is still limited, some evidence suggests that these therapies may provide additional benefits when used in conjunction with traditional approaches.

Acupuncture is an ancient Chinese medicine therapy that involves inserting thin needles into specific points on the body. Some studies suggest that acupuncture may have positive effects in treating insomnia, helping to regulate sleep and reduce anxiety. Acupuncture is believed to stimulate the central nervous system, promoting energy balance in the body. However, more research is needed to fully understand its mechanisms of action and effectiveness.

Chiropractic is a therapeutic approach that focuses on manipulating the spine and musculoskeletal system to improve overall health. Although chiropractic is not directly aimed at treating sleep or mental health, some patients report indirect benefits such as pain relief, muscle relaxation and improved general well-being. However, it is important to highlight that chiropractic does not replace conventional medical treatment and must be performed by a qualified professional.

Music therapy uses music as a therapeutic tool to promote relaxation, reduce anxiety and improve sleep. Music has the power to affect our emotions and moods, and many people find that listening to soft, calming music before bed can help induce sleep and create a peaceful environment. In addition, some relaxation techniques, such as binaural music or nature sounds, can be used to help induce sleep. Music therapy can be performed individually or with the guidance of a music therapist.

It's important to point out that while these complementary therapies may be beneficial for some people, not all approaches work for everyone. It is recommended to consult a qualified health professional, such as a doctor, a specialized therapist or a music therapist, for personalized and safe guidance.

***

Sleep quality plays a key role in mental health and there is a bidirectional relationship between the two. When sleep is compromised, either through deprivation or sleep disturbances, it can have a significant impact on mental health. On the other hand, mental disorders such as anxiety, depression and chronic stress can negatively affect the quality and duration of sleep.

Lack of adequate sleep can lead to changes in mood regulation, emotional processing, and the ability to handle stress. Chronic sleep deprivation is associated with a higher risk of developing mental disorders such as anxiety and depression. Furthermore, sleep disorders such as insomnia, sleep apnea and restless legs syndrome are often found in individuals with mental disorders, increasing the complexity of the clinical picture.

Therefore, it is crucial to address both sleep disorders and mental disorders in an integrated way. It is important to seek appropriate treatment for comorbid sleep disorders in cases of mental disorders in order to improve quality of life and promote recovery of mental health.

An effective approach to treating comorbid sleep disorders and supporting mental health is Cognitive Behavioral Therapy for Insomnia (CBT-I). CBT-I is an evidence-based therapy that aims to restructure the thought and behavior patterns that contribute to insomnia. It involves sleep reeducation techniques, stimulus control, sleep restriction and relaxation techniques, among other strategies. CBT-I has been shown to be effective in improving sleep quality and treating symptoms of anxiety and depression associated with insomnia.

In addition to CBT-I, meditation practices, mindfulness and other complementary therapies can also play an important role in promoting mental health through sleep. Meditation, for example, has been linked to significant benefits in reducing anxiety, stress and improving sleep. The practice of mindfulness, which involves being consciously present in the present moment, can help calm the mind and reduce rumination, thus facilitating relaxation and sleep induction.

Other complementary therapies such as acupuncture, yoga, aromatherapy and breathing techniques can also be helpful in improving sleep quality and promoting mental health. These approaches can help reduce stress, anxiety, and muscle tension, contributing to more restful sleep and an overall state of well-being.

However, it is important to emphasize that these complementary therapies should be used as part of a comprehensive treatment plan and under the guidance of qualified professionals. Each individual is unique and may respond differently to different therapeutic approaches. Therefore, it is essential to seek adequate and personalized guidance to determine which strategies are most suitable for each specific case.

In summary, recognizing the importance of sleep quality for mental health and seeking adequate treatment for comorbid sleep disorders in cases of mental disorders are essential steps to promote mental health. In addition, strategies such as CBT-I, meditation, mindfulness and other complementary therapies can be effective in improving mental health through sleep.

# The Role of the Dream

*The importance of dreams for health and emotional processing*

<u>understanding dreams</u>

Dreams are mental experiences that occur during sleep and involve a variety of elements such as images, emotions and narratives. They can range from vivid and memorable dreams to fragments of images and sensations. Dreams can be simple or complex, realistic or surreal, and often have a distinctly different quality to reality.

Dreams perform several important functions. One is emotional processing. During sleep, the brain has the opportunity to reprocess and deal with emotions experienced during the day. Dreams provide a safe space for emotional expression and conflict resolution, allowing the mind to work through stressful experiences, traumas or worries.

In addition, dreams also play a role in memory consolidation. During sleep, the brain revisits and reorganizes the information and experiences experienced throughout the day. Dreams can help with the selection and storage of important memories, making it easier to learn and retain information.

Dreams have also been linked to cognitive development. During REM sleep (Rapid Eye Movement, in English), the phase in which the most vivid dreams occur, there is an increase in brain activity related to visual processing, creative thinking and problem solving. It is believed that dreams can stimulate creativity, provide insights and facilitate the solution of complex problems.

While fully understanding the meaning of dreams remains a challenge, they remain a fascinating topic for scientific research and a source of inspiration for art and culture. Dream interpretation has been explored throughout history, with various theories and psychological approaches being proposed to understand its symbolism and potential personal meaning.

It is important to highlight that dreams are individual and personal experiences. They reflect the unique interplay between each individual's mind, life experiences and emotions. Although there are common patterns and themes in dreams, the interpretation of each dream must be considered in the personal and subjective context of each person.

In short, dreams are rich and complex mental experiences that occur during sleep. They play a key role in emotional processing, memory consolidation and cognitive development. Although their exact function is still the subject of study, dreams provide a window into the inner world of the human mind and have continued to fascinate and intrigue people throughout the ages.

## emotional processing

Dreams play an important role in emotional processing, providing a safe and creative space to express and process intense or repressed feelings. During sleep, the brain has the opportunity to reactivate emotionally charged memories and integrate them in a healthy way, facilitating the regulation of emotional responses.

One of the mechanisms involved in emotional processing during sleep is the reactivation of memories. During dreams, the brain can reactivate emotionally significant memories, allowing these experiences to be relived and symbolically reprocessed. This can help to reduce the emotional intensity associated with past events and facilitate the assimilation and understanding of past experiences.

Furthermore, dreams provide a safe context for the expression and release of pent-up emotions. During sleep, the restrictions and inhibitions that are normally imposed during wakefulness are lessened. This allows intense or repressed feelings to be experienced and expressed more freely and creatively in dreams. This emotional release can help relieve built-up emotional tension and promote healthy emotional balance.

Dreams are also involved in regulating emotional responses. During REM sleep, when the most vivid dreams occur, there is increased activity in the limbic system, which is responsible for emotions. This activity can help regulate and balance emotional responses, providing an opportunity for the brain to process and integrate the emotional experiences of the previous day.

It is important to point out that emotional processing in dreams is not always direct or literal. The emotions and content of dreams can be symbolic or metaphorical, reflecting how the mind deals with emotions and personal experiences. Therefore, the interpretation of dreams must be considered within the individual context of each person.

In short, dreams play a crucial role in emotional processing, providing a safe space for expressing and processing intense or repressed feelings. Through reactivation of memories, emotional release and regulation of emotional responses, dreams assist in the healthy integration of emotional experiences and contribute to emotional balance and mental well-being.

### adaptive dream function

Dreams also play an adaptive role, as they can help with problem solving, rehearsing situations, and processing traumatic events. Through dreams, the brain has the ability to simulate different scenarios and experiences, which can be beneficial for survival and personal development.

One of the adaptive functions of dreams is problem solving. During sleep, the brain continues to work on issues and challenges faced during the day. Dreams can provide an environment where you can explore different solutions and perspectives without the limitations and restrictions of the real world. This ability to process information and find new approaches can contribute to creativity, decision making and problem solving.

Dreams can also play a role in rehearsing situations. For example, in vivid, realistic dreams, you can practice fine motor skills or rehearse social and emotional scenarios. This can help improve performance in specific activities and develop soft skills. Dreams offer a safe environment to experiment with different possibilities and learn from experiences.

Additionally, dreams have been linked to processing traumatic events. During sleep, the brain has the ability to revisit and process emotionally disturbing memories in a controlled manner. This can help assimilate and reorganize these experiences, contributing to emotional recovery and resilience.

From an evolutionary perspective, there are theories that suggest that dreams have adaptive advantages. One such theory is the behavioral assay hypothesis, which postulates that dreams can help individuals prepare for future challenges. For example, dreaming of resolving social conflicts can help develop negotiation and cooperation skills.

Another theory is the emotional processing hypothesis, which suggests that dreams play a role in emotion regulation and the consolidation of emotional memory. Dreams allow emotions to be experienced and processed in a safe and controlled way, contributing to emotional balance and adaptation to lived experiences.

While these theories provide interesting insights into the adaptive function of dreams, it is important to note that the study of dreams is still ongoing and there is no definitive consensus on their exact functions. Dreams are complex and multifaceted phenomena, and understanding their adaptive function continues to be the subject of research and debate.

In short, dreams perform an adaptive function, allowing for problem solving, rehearsing situations, and processing traumatic events. Through dreams, the brain can explore different possibilities, practice skills and deal with intense emotions. While evolutionary theories suggest that dreams may have evolved to provide adaptive advantages, a full understanding of their adaptive function is still under development.

## *Dream interpretation: psychological and cultural approaches*

### psychological approaches

Psychological approaches offer different perspectives on dream interpretation and can provide insights into the symbolic meaning and content of dreams. Two widely known theories are Sigmund Freud's psychoanalytic theory and the cognitive-behavioral theory of dreams.

Freud's psychoanalytic theory suggests that dreams are symbolic expressions of unconscious desires and repressed emotions.

According to this theory, dreams are a manifestation of the process of wishing and wish-fulfillment, which occurs during sleep. Freud believed that dreams are a form of symbolic expression of unconscious desires and impulses that cannot be freely expressed in conscious life. He argued that dreams have both manifest content (what is remembered) and latent content (the actual symbolic meaning). Dream interpretation involves unraveling the symbolic meaning underlying dream elements, which can provide insights into the individual's unconscious conflicts and desires.

Cognitive-behavioral dream theory, on the other hand, focuses on the adaptive function of dreams and information processing during sleep. This approach emphasizes the importance of cognitive processes in the formation of dreams.

According to this theory, dreams are a way of processing and organizing information and experiences from the previous day. Dreams reflect the individual's cognitive and emotional activities, such as thoughts, concerns and lived experiences. Dream interpretation in the cognitive-behavioral approach focuses on understanding how dream elements are related to the individual's experiences and cognitive processes.

Both approaches make significant contributions to the understanding of dreams, albeit with different approaches. The psychoanalytic approach highlights the importance of the unconscious and symbolic contents of dreams, while the cognitive-behavioral approach focuses on the cognitive and adaptive processes involved in dreams. It is important to emphasize that dream interpretation is not an exact science, and different perspectives can coexist.

In addition to these theories, there are other psychological approaches that explore the meaning of dreams, such as the humanistic approach, which emphasizes self-realization and personal growth, and the transpersonal approach, which seeks to understand the spiritual and transcendental dimension of dreams.

## cultural influence

Cultural influence plays a significant role in dream interpretation. Cultural beliefs, values, and symbols can shape the understanding and interpretation of dreams in unique ways across different societies and communities.

Each culture has its own traditions, myths and meanings attributed to dreams. For example, in some indigenous cultures, dreams are considered to be important spiritual messages or premonitions. In contrast, in certain contemporary Western cultures, dreams can be seen more as personal and symbolic expressions of the individual psyche.

Symbols and meanings attributed to dream elements can also vary culturally. A given symbol or image may have different interpretations in different cultures. For example, a specific animal might be considered sacred in one culture, while in another culture, it might be seen as a symbol of bad luck.

Furthermore, experiences and cultural contexts influence how dreams are interpreted. Life experiences, family traditions, and cultural norms shape each individual's understanding of dreams. For example, a recurring dream about marriage might be interpreted differently by a person living in a culture that highly values marriage compared to someone from a culture that places less emphasis on this institution.

It is important to consider the cultural context when interpreting dreams meaningfully. Dream interpretation must take into account prevailing cultural beliefs and values, as well as each person's individual experience and personal associations. Interpreting dreams in a broader cultural context can help provide a richer and more complete understanding of their meaning.

While culture can provide context and influence interpretation, it is the individual perspective that gives meaning to dreams. Therefore, it is important for each person to explore and reflect on their own dreams, taking into account both cultural influence and personal experience.

## *Techniques for remembering and recording dreams meaningfully*

Improving dream recall

Improving dream recall can be an interesting practice for those who wish to explore their dream world more deeply. There are some strategies that can be useful in this regard:

**Keeping a Dream Journal:** Keeping a dream journal next to your bed is an effective practice for recording your dreams right after waking up. Upon waking up, try to remember as many details of the dream as possible and write them down in your diary. Include information such as characters, settings, emotions, and significant events. Writing immediately after waking helps to fix dream memories before they fade into memory.

**Intention before going to sleep:** Before going to sleep, say positive affirmations or visualize yourself remembering your dreams when you wake up. Reinforcing the intention to remember dreams can have a positive impact on your ability to recall them. Tell yourself that you will remember the dreams and that they will be vivid and clear.

**Scheduled awakenings:** Set your alarm clock to go off during a sleep period when you are most likely to be in a REM (rapid eye movement) sleep phase, which is when the most vivid dreams occur. When you wake up during or just after a period of REM sleep, you are more likely to remember your dreams. Immediately write down any dreams you recall.

**Maintain a peaceful environment when waking up:** When waking up, try to lie still for a few minutes before getting up. Staying in a peaceful, relaxed environment can help preserve dream memories before they dissipate.

In addition to these suggestions, it is interesting to point out that overall sleep quality can also affect dream recall. Good sleep hygiene, including creating an environment conducive to sleep, practicing relaxation techniques before bed, and maintaining a regular sleep schedule, can contribute to more restful sleep and better dream recall.

Remembering dreams can be an enriching experience, allowing for greater understanding of oneself, emotional processing and creativity. By applying these strategies, you can increase your ability to remember and explore dreams, tapping into the insights and imagination they can provide.

## Exploring and interpreting dreams

Exploring and interpreting dreams can be a fascinating journey of self-discovery and emotional understanding. Here are some guidelines to help you analyze and interpret your dreams:

**Identify key elements:** When reviewing your dreams, pay attention to key elements such as people, objects, places and situations. They can play a significant role in dream interpretation. Write down all the important details that you remember.

**Notice recurring patterns:** If you notice recurring patterns in your dreams, such as specific themes, situations or symbols, this could indicate the presence of underlying issues or emotions in your life. Try to identify these patterns and explore what they might mean to you.

**Connect with your emotions:** When analyzing your dreams, note the emotions you felt during the dream and those that persist after waking up. Emotions awakened by dreams can provide valuable clues about your deepest concerns, desires or fears. Consider how these emotions relate to your daily life and recent events.

**Explore personal symbols:** Dreams can be filled with personal symbols that have unique meaning for you. These symbols can vary from person to person, so it's important to consider your personal associations with certain symbols. Ask yourself what these symbols mean to you and how they relate to your life experience.

**Keep a dream journal:** Keeping a dream journal can be a valuable tool to help you analyze and interpret your dreams over time. Write down your dreams regularly, including details, emotions, and any insights or reflections you may have. As you review your journal, you may notice recurring patterns and themes that will help you better understand the meaning of your dreams.

If you wish to explore the meaning of your dreams more deeply, consider consulting a professional, such as a therapist who specializes in dream analysis or analytical psychology. They can provide additional perspective and help you explore the symbolic and emotional aspects of your dreams in a deeper way.

Dreams can be rich in personal and emotional insights, exploration and interpretation of dreams can be a valuable tool for self-knowledge, reflection and personal growth.

## Incorporating dreams into the personal journey

Incorporating dreams into your personal journey can be a powerful way to harness the potential for self-awareness and personal growth they offer. Here are some suggestions for exploring dreams as a significant source of insight and learning:

**Working with therapists who specialize in dream interpretation:** Therapists specializing in dream interpretation can help to deepen understanding of the symbolic meanings of dreams and to explore the emotional and psychological aspects associated with them.

They can provide a professional perspective and guide you on your journey of self-exploration through dreams.

**Participate in dream discussion groups:** Participating in dream discussion groups or dream circles can be an enriching way to share and explore dream experiences with others. These groups provide a safe space to share dreams, exchange different insights and perspectives, and learn from others' experiences. Collaborating and interacting with other people interested in dreams can further enrich your own understanding of dreams.

**Personal reflection and integration:** Take time to reflect on the dreams you remember and consider the messages, emotions and insights they may convey. Write down your dreams and do a personal analysis, connecting them with your everyday life, past events, relationships and personal challenges. Ask yourself how dreams can offer new perspectives, guidance or solutions to issues you are facing.

**Creative practices:** In addition to personal reflection, you can explore your dreams through creative practices such as writing stories, creating art, or expressing yourself through dance or music. These practices can help access the emotions and insights evoked by dreams in a more intuitive and expressive way, allowing for a deeper understanding of their personal meaning.

***

Dreams play a significant role in mental health, emotional processing and personal development. Here are some points to highlight their importance:

**Mental health:** Dreams have an intrinsic connection with our mental health. They offer a window into our deepest thoughts and emotions, allowing us to express and process aspects of our psyche that may not be accessible in our waking state. By exploring dreams, we can gain insights into our fears, desires, traumas and concerns, contributing to a better understanding of ourselves and strengthening our mental health.

**Emotional processing:** Dreams play a key role in emotional processing. During sleep, the brain reactivates and revisits emotional memories and experiences, allowing us to safely process and integrate these emotions. Dreams offer an opportunity to express, symbolize and regulate intense or repressed emotions, assisting in the resolution of emotional conflicts and emotional balance.

**Personal development:** Dreams can play a vital role in our personal development. By reflecting on the themes, symbols, and narratives of dreams, we can gain insights into our deepest desires, goals, and aspirations. Dreams can offer us guidance and inspiration, helping us to explore new paths, overcome challenges and develop personal skills. They can be a source of creativity, intuition and self-awareness, providing valuable resources for personal growth and development.

**Psychological and cultural perspectives:** Dream interpretation can be approached from different psychological and cultural perspectives. Theories such as Freud's psychoanalysis, the cognitive-behavioral approach, and humanistic psychology offer different lenses for understanding dreams. Also, different cultures have specific traditions and interpretations for dreams, with unique symbols and meanings. It is important to recognize that dream interpretation is highly personal and may vary according to each individual's perspective and cultural background.

**Practices for remembering and exploring dreams:** To take full advantage of the benefits of dreams, it is helpful to adopt practices that enhance dream recall and exploration. Keeping a dream journal next to your bed and recording your dreams as soon as you wake up is an effective way to capture the images and emotions you experience. Also, setting an intention before bed to remember your dreams and practicing personal reflection on the content and meaning of your dreams helps you gain valuable insights into yourself.

By encouraging the practice of dream exploration, we are promoting self-awareness, creativity and personal development. Dreams offer fertile ground for discovering our inner world, allowing us to expand our understanding of ourselves and the symbolic universe we inhabit. By dedicating time and attention to dreams, we can benefit from their wisdom and harness their transformative power.

# Conclusion

Throughout this work, we explore the various aspects of sleep and dreams, highlighting their importance for mental health, emotional well-being and personal development. We learned about the importance of good sleep hygiene, creating an environment conducive to rest, and implementing relaxing practices before bed. We also discuss the effects of sleep deprivation, comorbid sleep disorders, and therapeutic approaches to promoting healthy sleep.

It became clear that sleep plays a key role in our mental and emotional health. A good quality of sleep is essential for the regulation of emotions, memory consolidation, emotional processing and the general balance of our well-being. In addition, dreams provide us with deep access to our inner world, allowing us to explore our desires, fears, desires and emotions in a unique way.

As we better understand the relationship between sleep, dreams and mental health, it becomes clear that we must prioritize adequate sleep and adopt practices that promote healthy sleep. From infancy to old age, each stage of life presents specific sleep challenges, and it's important to adapt our strategies to meet our needs at each stage.

At the same time, we recognize that each individual is unique, and finding personalized approaches to improving sleep and exploring dreams is essential. We can experiment with different techniques, such as cognitive behavioral therapy, meditation, mindfulness, complementary therapies, and individual dream exploration, to find what works best for us.

Therefore, in concluding this work, it is evident that sleep and dreams play a crucial role in our health and well-being. By prioritizing quality sleep, adopting relaxation practices, and exploring dream insights, we can promote emotional balance, deeper self-awareness, and meaningful personal growth. It is an invitation for each of us to embrace the power of sleep and dreams in our journey towards a full and healthy life.

Printed in Great Britain
by Amazon